THE KEEPER OF THE STORIES

THE KEEPER OF THE STORIES

*Tales from a Life in Medicine
Years Spent Tilting at Windmills*

MICHAEL LEVIN, MD

Copyright © 2015 by Michael Levin, MD.

Library of Congress Control Number: 2015912347
ISBN: Hardcover   978-1-5035-9173-8
            Softcover   978-1-5035-9172-1
            eBook   978-1-5035-9171-4

All rights reserved. No part of this book may be reproduced or transmitted in any form or by any means, electronic or mechanical, including photocopying, recording, or by any information storage and retrieval system, without permission in writing from the copyright owner.

Any people depicted in stock imagery provided by Thinkstock are models, and such images are being used for illustrative purposes only.
Certain stock imagery © Thinkstock.

Print information available on the last page.

Rev. date: 09/17/2015

To order additional copies of this book, contact:
Xlibris
1-888-795-4274
www.Xlibris.com
Orders@Xlibris.com
715338

This book is dedicated to the memory of my parents, Arnold and Elaine Levin; to my children Anna, Dan, Ben and his wife Allison; especially to my wife Terry and our wonderful granddaughter, Catherine Virginia Levin.

Not every book requires acknowledgements, but this one does. Thank you Rudolph Hardy, Max Arbeiter and Lee Suyemoto— all of whom insisted that I finish this book. Thanks to the San Francisco Examiner for allowing me to reproduce their articles and photos. Thanks to Rose Aprigian, Michael Weil, Erica Schwartrz, Tamar Neuman, the Collela family, Hans Hinteregger, Anna Marx, Eric Marmorek, Thelma Vasil, Robert Fiske, Jan Brodau, and the many patients who I've been privileged to treat. I add Jerome Ludwig who knows what he's talking about. Nick Browning (Sancho Panza), Jeff Alexander, Sue Katz, Christine Stone and Clem Van Buren who provided advice along the way. My children Ben, Dan, and Anna who not only transcribed, but provided precious input. And to Terry, who provided everything else.

If history were taught in the form of stories, it would never be forgotten.

—Rudyard Kipling

CONTENTS

The Health-Care Morass 1
Medicine 6
A Great Save 9
Medicine: Many Years Before The Save 15

MEDICAL SCHOOL

The First Time 27
Percent 31
Media 34
The Urinal 37

INTENSIVE CARE UNIT AND SOME OUTPATIENT CARE

Alcohol 40
Turning Yellow 44
Phosphorus 47
Expectations 50
Beauty 52
Lateness 56
A Lesson 59
Regret 62

OFFICE

Chance First Meeting..70
The Stamp Collector's Family 82
Losing Words..88
Tattoo 92
Apology..102
The Man Who Met Hitler And Einstein....................104
Inspiration..110
Camp 114
The Role Of Writing..117
Alliances 121
Poetry 130
Mental Health..137
Therapy..140
Vulnerability 142
Transition...144
International 147
To Do Good 150
Trip To Mexico 156
Octopus Trap 159
The Last Time 161
The Trap?...164
The Last Word 167

Don't think you can't learn something about human nature from rodents. In 2011, a study looking at the capacity for kindness among rats emerged from the University of Chicago. In the study, thirty rats were housed as fifteen pairs with each pair sharing the same cage for two weeks in order to become familiar with each other. After two weeks, the couples were separated, and one of the two rats was placed in a transparent glass cylinder lodged within a larger cage. Trapped within that cylinder, it was unable to escape. The second rat was introduced into the cage but was allowed to run freely and with abandon. The restrained rat in the glass cylinder would squeal and try in vain to escape. The "free" rat would desperately try to liberate the trapped rat by gnawing on the glass cylinder and, with a seeming sense of urgency, by frantically pulling the confined rats tail that protruded from the trap. This was not what the scientists expected. Eventually, the free rat discovered a lever, which opened a door that would result in freeing the trapped rat. Once the free rat figured this out, it used the lever to liberate the trapped rat immediately whenever it was reintroduced into the cage. This behavior was consistent for all the couples. This was not reported to occur in rats that had not been previously paired up, implying the need to know each other in order to help each other.

Next, the experimenters put stuffed fake rats in the same restraint system, but the free rat would not push the lever to release the fake rat like they would a buddy.

In another twist, the free rats would open the door for the trapped rats even if that only resulted in those rats being released into a different cage, thus discounting any assumption that the release was solely the selfish desire for companionship, but rather indicating that the purpose of the release was to end the distress of the other rat.

Finally, the researchers added a pile of chocolate chips to a corner of the cage (rats love chocolate) and found that the free rat would still release the trapped rat even though it meant sharing the cherished chocolate.

Noting similar findings among the fifteen pairs of rats, the scientists concluded that compassion and empathy are inherited traits that have evolved in rat DNA and, presumably, in other mammals, like us.

And, I think, that's why there are firemen, teachers, social workers, nurses, relief organizations, and doctors. Social networks can influence us as human beings are "paired" together. Perhaps through our "primed" DNA, we already have the capacity for empathy and compassion, which is the hallmark of humanity. It must be nurtured and developed to get to the point where we are selfless. For an internist, our inherent traits are enhanced by interaction with our patients, many of whom we remember over a lifetime.

But DNA can mutate. We all have the potential to disorder our empathy and compassion, as you will see.

In autumn of 2011, I was contacted by the concerned daughter and son-in-law of my patient Ethel C. Ethel was eighty-eight, suffering from mild dementia and, in spite of using a walker, was having extreme difficulty ambulating. Three months earlier, while living in New York City, she had fallen and had fractured her right hip. At a local New York hospital, she underwent surgical repair and then moved to Boston in order to be cared for by her daughter and son-in-law.

When they called, I was told that Ethel's left forearm was red and swollen and looked infected. Her family was concerned that this was why she wouldn't use the walker and was not walking. She was taken to the emergency room where an arm infection was diagnosed and an X-ray revealed a newly fractured hip near the region of the previously repaired hip fracture. She had probably fallen but had not mentioned it because of her dementia or, possibly, because of a deeply embedded fear of losing further control and freedom. She was admitted to the hospital, and an orthopedic surgeon was consulted. He advised surgery, but initially she refused. Perhaps she feared she would become further confined. The medical resident now felt there was nothing more we could offer beyond care for the arm infection.

The following day, her arm was better, but Ethel remained in bed. In spite of attempts to get her to move, she refused. I assumed this was due to pain and difficulty related to her newly refractured hip, but she did not explain her recalcitrance. Since she had refused surgery, the case manager (a nurse hired by the hospital to ensure that patients don't spend costly extra days in the hospital—the case manager is given a prominent role in the hospital bureaucracy in order to advise the doctor about the cost of prolonged, poorly reimbursed hospital stays, which may benefit the hospital bottom line at the expense of patient welfare) decided Ethel should be sent home. I asked whether she could be sent to a temporary rehab facility instead of home while we tried to sort out the surgical situation, but I was told that insurance coverage for rehab requires a three-day hospital stay.

"So," I said, "let's keep her for three days."

"We can't," replied the nurse/case manager.

"But she can't walk," I countered.

"Yes, she can," answered the crafty nurse.

I was incredulous. "How do you know this?"

"Because she told me," the nurse responded triumphantly.

"But she has dementia," I blurted.

I noticed that Ethel had developed an abnormal heart rhythm. Her heart had switched from normal sinus rhythm to atrial fibrillation. The nurse/case manager called over the medical resident, who stated with supreme confidence that the rhythm was not atrial fibrillation and that the patient could be discharged.

Although it is possible to misread a heart rhythm, there are fairly simple ways of examining an EKG and clarifying the problem, but that approach wasn't done immediately. Apparently, she too was under pressure from the case manager to discharge the patient, and that would have the extra benefit of reducing her own workload. She did not take the time to adequately assess the EKG. I wasn't used to this new system whereby the cost pressure, as represented by the case manager, is placed on equal footing with the medical decisions determined by the patient's physician.

As they walked off, I made one last plea for my patient. Had they seen the tattoo on Ethel's left forearm? It was a number, and it was often that number that Ethel would recite when referring to herself, "I'm 15744." It was placed on her forearm at Auschwitz/Buchenwald during World War II. They each responded that they had noticed it. Nothing seemed to impact their hope to discharge Ethel against my wishes.

It is clear that the cost of care is higher for the very ill and that we will suffer more illness as we age, and though technology is available to prolong life, the resources are limited. The doctor who knows their patient is in the best position to evaluate the viability of their patient and the types of interventions that make sense.

I then walked away, paged the cardiologist on call, and asked her to come by and interpret the EKG, which she immediately interpreted as atrial fibrillation. I asked her to discuss it with the medical resident, who later apologized to me and explained how case management has focused on patient discharge with the unfortunate consequence of blurring the real needs of the patient and the judgment of fledgling doctors.

Ethel stayed for three days, went to rehab, and returned at the end of the week for surgery. She was now back with her daughter and son-in-law and walking with a walker—she was freed from confinement. The case manager barely spoke to me. The head of the hospital informed me that cases like this result in reduced revenue for the hospital, and I could be more circumspect. So I wrote this book.

THE HEALTH-CARE MORASS

Hello, you've reached your insurer. How may we thwart you?

In 1993 the nation expected the Clinton administration to radically change health-care delivery in the United States. My involvement was limited to a few small-group meetings at the Old Executive Building and at the White House. The assembled group included about twenty doctors from around the country and members of the administration. Many doctors and patients were thrilled with the possibility of universal health care while others expressed doubt compounded by a fear of the unknown. The first lady was painted a socialist and harridan. Vituperative attacks abounded, regaling the populace about how a national health-care program would work like the postal service. (I kept thinking how I get my mail delivered rain, sleet, or snow every day except Sundays and holidays and how I take that for granted—not socialism, but a social service.) Medicare remained a single-party payer for those over sixty-five, and it worked until perverse Republican and Democratic regulations drastically restricted care on our most vulnerable members of society (the legislators and lobbyists luxuriating in their triumph). Debate raged, and there was a powerful impetus to create affordable, government-administered universal health care, but it was not easy. Much of the dialogue was introduced by the auto industry, which had fallen on hard times in the 1970s and laid off many workers.

Profits were praised with starry-eyed adoration even as jobs were lost. (They were harbingers of Enron, Lehman Brothers, AIG, subprime lending, Goldman Sachs, and the fiasco of the financial collapse of 2008—companies filled with hardheaded executives who felt they could see the world as it really is.)

In Detroit, the auto industry had improved manufacturing technology to the extent that they could rid themselves of now-redundant workers. As part of the deal with the autoworkers union, an agreement had been hammered out to provide health care for laid-off and retired workers. That news filled the air while I was a medical student in Detroit, yet few thought that the cost of medical care was particularly outrageous—indeed, the US health system was considered the paradigm of world medical care, something few suggest today.

Twenty years later, during the Clinton health-care debate, technology had expanded exponentially, and great health benefits were enjoyed by most of the populace, but at enormous costs. This is why insurance reform became a primary issue for Bill Clinton when he took over the White House. Disturbingly, special interests and corporate mentality, particularly those of the insurance companies, ruled the day, and the plan failed as enormous, obscene profits for the insurance industry increased.

In a front-page *Wall Street Journal* article, an insurance executive said that the Clinton administration tried to involve managed-care companies in health-care reform, but instead the involvement of profit-oriented insurers was "the goose that laid the golden egg." Like the ingestion of caustic lye burning through from inside out, the insurers thrived on the caustic lie that they put patient care above corporate profits, burning through health-care dollars from the inside out. We are now left trying to pick up the pieces of a decimated system without losing the essence of medicine. What seemed lost in the debate was the relationship between the doctor and the patient. Medicare has now been adulterated to the extent that a post office analogy seems apropos. It's as if the daily mail were picked up, the letter opened and read by a postal worker who then decides whether the letter warrants a higher-priced stamp, makes some alterations to the text, or perhaps determines that the letter shouldn't be sent at all.

Albert Camus wrote, "When one has no character one has to apply a method." The health-care industry has been so driven by profits that talk of character seems naive, quaint even. What is truly naive is that doctors in the primary-care fields have been discouraged by these changes, and there is now a desperate attempt to fill the void. Fewer medical students want to enter primary care. Primary-care fields have always garnered less pay, but medical students flocked into those fields because of the belief that they would have a positive impact on a patient's life. An experienced doctor knew, with little doubt, the enemy (disease) and how to most efficiently mount an attack. It was the variety of cases, the interaction with patients, and the feeling of autonomy that led to enthusiastic medical students entering primary-care fields. We listen to the patient gossip and even learn a bit of history in the process. Now very few medical students are aware of the virtues of being a person's primary doctor. That, in turn, prompts the question, Has the doctor become so co-opted or disillusioned that he or she will no longer find passion and commitment in his or her work and, a priori, the patient? Can we lose sight of the health requirements of the most needy, the poor, and the elderly who are getting hustled toward managed-care companies in order to maintain or reapportion profits? Does a patient have no value unless they render a financial reward?

As I began listening and collecting stories, a sea change was occurring in medicine. Managed-care plans were beginning to take hold, and they made profits by restricting diagnostic tests and treatments. The numbers of health-care administrators rose relative to the numbers of doctors. Those were sudden, unanticipated changes, and many doctors and patients were dissatisfied. Fewer and fewer medical students were choosing to go into the field of internal medicine in part because of less exposure to role models. Hospitalists (doctors hired by the hospital to see patients in the hospital, but not before or after hospitalization) replaced private doctors in the hospital setting, with strong doctor-patient relationships slipping through the cracks. Doctors were dropping out of the field as they became discouraged with less autonomy as more restrictions were created by managed-care companies and insurance networks (companies focused on the bottom line, not unlike any moneymaking business). Something insidious was happening. Computers were used for record keeping and communication (not a bad idea and in many ways enhancing aspects of patient care, but it resulted in less doctor-to-doctor conversation and interaction—I can think of innumerable cases where telephone conversations with other doctors saved a life or made a remarkable diagnosis). And in order to maximize payments for insurers, electronic medical records (incorporating information and often misinformation) were mandated and could result in institutionalized fraud because you will be paid less unless you enhance the record according to the insurer's code system. Often those entering data into records have an eye on remuneration and not necessarily on good patient care.

The slide away from responsibility has been easier than we thought as fear can cause us to ignore our better instincts. Presently we are told to be afraid of many things: the high cost of medicine and any government system planning to tax and spend us to oblivion. When it comes to medicine, we have been warned, in dire terms, that runaway medical costs will ruin us. "Beware of Medicare" is the mantra most repeated by insurance executives. But opposing the insidious monster of fear, Medicare has done more to protect our elderly than anything private health care has offered. They say that Medicare will result in rationing, but what is it called when managed-care companies restrict access to certain medications, procedures, and treatments?

Over the past thirty years, in order to "perfect" medical care, the numbers of insurance administrators and bureaucrats have increased exponentially while the numbers of doctors per population has remained relatively flat. The insurers and their health-care alliances reassure us that they will protect us from such governmental destruction (and take a little off the top for themselves, like the operator of a hedge fund). With marketing and administrative costs, "off the top" can run from 10 to 30 percent—the pleasure of reaping financial rewards at the expense of those in need. This schadenfreude results in enormous profits for health-care companies but at the same time creates multiple bureaucratic restrictions, reducing incentives for doctors to practice "primary care."

The stories in this collection give the reader a glimpse into the learning process of a physician and how experience teaches all of us. Until now, in accordance with the precepts of Hippocrates, the practice of medicine had been divorced from the business model. It is the patient's fear, with good reason, that the physician will succumb to the pressure that the insurers bring to bear; the concern is that the medical establishment has lost sight of the mission and is no longer the ethical beacon it once was. Fledgling doctors are concerned that the passion of the physician will get stamped out. I would hope that these stories speak to some of those concerns and reestablish a patient-oriented focus.

Twenty years ago almost all doctors were satisfied with their profession. Now that number is less than 10 percent. Polls of doctors indicate dissatisfaction with computer records—and for good reason. They report both inefficiency and reduced quality of care. Who benefits from unhappy doctors?

MEDICINE

Why Aren't There Enough Doctors?

At a medical conference, a revered physician rises and addresses the audience, "I am among the front line of doctors as insurance and computer mandates are instituted, and I feel like one of the soldiers in the first wave landing at Normandy, slaughtered by machine gunfire. To the left, they retire; to the right, they leave for concierge medicine. I am overwhelmed, so that's why I'm reluctantly retiring."

One blurry-eyed colleague moans, "I'm ready to give up. I hate the mandated computer system with the Byzantine codes. We're told that entering data takes precedence over a dying patient and that following an algorithm should replace the thought process we've developed by years of experience. The computer freezes, breaks down, and when it malfunctions, as it does with regularity, we find we can't think without it."

"I imagine the sickly, sweet, yet grim smile of the insurance executives," says another, "as they rake in profits while denying care, not answering appeal requests, and always referring us to electronic menus that lead to dead ends or someplace in Bangalore. We're not told which tests are covered or even if they'll pay for prescription medications. The insurers seem disturbed to have to deal with a health delivery system that involves doctors or sick patients. How mad are we expected to get? Worse yet, what will happen when we stop getting mad?"

"I can't take the bureaucracy, the morass of insurance restrictions," complains an older internist. "We are unable to provide appropriate care even if they have insurance. And we are under economic pressure to reduce care to the elderly. They say that if our patients are hospitalized longer than the Medicare insurance reviewer allows, we will be financially punished. In the face of the inordinate expectations, I should consider boutique medicine."

Sitting with a group of doctors, I've heard a series of complaints: "We've been coerced to join hospital networks that are part of insurance conglomerates. They've added thousands of administrators and multitudes of computer systems to cut costs—what horse manure! These large health networks intend to go public, answering only to investors and bondholders. Once employed, we are given Hobson's choice as we are forbidden to put patient concerns above company profits for fear of losing our jobs. Disgruntled physicians can't be good for the health of anyone."

"Interns, residents, and hospitalists are told that in order to meet metrics, they must enter very specific data into the computer, try to discharge patients as rapidly as possible, and that it's not necessary to spend the time to know their patients well. This ensures that the future success of the insurance system is locked in because the interns and residents are pressured to be more responsive to computers and administrators than to their patients. We run the risk of making each previous generation obsolete." She shakes her head in disgust.

"When the computer went down, it was interesting, refreshing, and enjoyable. We started paying attention to our patients again and not to the screen. No one wants the doctor to be obligated to think this way. We forgot how to take responsibility for our patients. What's happened to us? The corporatization of medicine has crushed our enthusiasm for patient care," comments a young doctor, having lost interest in medical practice.

"The system inhibits doctors from following their patients in the hospital. We've assured distrust, which serves to remove the important role of the doctor-patient relationship in healing. Instead of that perverse system, I think that once the patient is hospitalized, their doctor should be formally consulted in order to provide continuity and reestablish trust. Hospitals and health plans don't permit the patient to request their own doctor to take care of them in the hospital, solely aiding hospital profit, not actual patient care!" notes a physician who was recently forced to turn his hospitalized patients over to the hospitalist system—part of a health-care network described as "an octopus without a soul."

Such comments are made on a regular basis. I hear it in the hospital corridors and on the medical wards and read it in opinion pieces in medical as well as lay literature. The result is that medical students are no longer flocking to primary-care practices, some even becoming health-care administrators in the perverse hope of avoiding the bureaucracy placed on the shoulders of practicing physicians. This is not simply a financial issue since the pay is not bad for most doctors. Medical students were once impressed by the sense of dedication and job satisfaction they saw in internists, and they chose to emulate those physicians. There was an intense feeling of responsibility for our patient's well-being. But life in medicine has fundamentally changed since the days when we would enthusiastically share the details of the most recent incredible case or share exhilarating stories about a great save.

A GREAT SAVE

The winters in New England can be quite bitter, and it's not unusual to hear a passerby rant that they're "sick of the cold." And so it was with Patrick.

In his early sixties, Patrick had hypertension and hyperlipidemia. He did well with medications and regular checkups. His routine had been predictable: oatmeal for breakfast, e-mail prospective clients for his job performing executive searches and sales, take the dog for a walk, complete the *New York Times* crossword puzzle, watch a bit of news, and perhaps meet someone about a business deal. Due to a precipitous dive in the economy, those meetings became less frequent, which gave him more opportunity to walk the dog in the freezing cold and maybe catch more of the news.

On this particular Thursday in January, US Airways flight 1549 emergency landed in the Hudson River with no loss of life, and media were filled with the heroics of the airplane personnel and Captain Sully Sullenberger's cool under pressure. However, Patrick never got a chance to hear anything about the event. Instead, while walking the dog in frigid weather outside his suburban Boston home, he noticed a squeezing pain in the middle of his chest. He took the dog home, looked up chest pain in his home medical reference manual, then drove up to the drugstore to pick up something for indigestion. On the way, he decided to call my office from his car. My secretary, Frances, told him to go right in, which he reluctantly agreed to do.

I was with a patient in an examining room when Patrick arrived in the already crowded waiting room. He had to wait a couple of minutes until the other exam room was freed up so that an EKG could be performed by Linda, the medical assistant, in order to evaluate his heart—to make certain that his chest discomfort had not been a symptom of an acute heart attack.

While waiting amid several other patients in my small, overflowing office, Patrick asked whether he might have a glass of water. Frances provided it, after which he said he felt fine, grabbed his coat, and notified Frances that he would be off. But Frances doesn't allow such behavior. Once you're within her jurisdiction, you're trapped there until she releases you.

"You can't go until the doctor sees you and looks at your EKG," she said. Within another minute, he was back in an examining room, hooked up for the EKG. The medical assistant said Patrick looked at the EKG after it came off the machine. He said it looked fine to him, so he would be leaving. I suppose that was an example of Patrick's irreverent sense of humor (at least that's what his wife now says, since he's a salesman, not a doctor, and has had absolutely no medical training).

Patrick didn't leave the examining room as he had threatened. Instead he got dressed and lay down on the examining table, which was where I found him when I entered the room. Just prior, I had looked at the EKG and noted the ominous peaked T waves of an acute anterior wall myocardial infarction. Before walking into the room, I yelled to Frances, "Call transport, stat," but then changed my mind: "No, it will take too long. Get a wheelchair and I'll wheel him over to the emergency room myself." Since the medical office building is attached to the hospital, I figured I'd save some time. I grabbed aspirin to give him, because that is standard early treatment for an acute heart attack, and I walked in.

Patrick was still wearing glasses. His gray hair was neatly cropped. He appeared trim and fit with his white shirt perfectly tucked into tan pleated trousers, lying on the examining table, fully dressed, blue and unresponsive—he was dead.

Actually, as Billy Crystal's character Miracle Max said in *The Princess Bride*, he was "just mostly dead."

Unable to arouse him, I began pumping on his chest, performing mouth-to-mouth resuscitation and shouting for Frances to call a code blue, which would prompt the hospital emergency code team to get over to help. In the meantime, one of my waiting-room patients mentioned that she worked for hospital security and said that just two weeks before, a code kit had been placed near the elevators on every floor of the medical building in an attempt to improve upon our limited ability to save lives due to the fact that most patients in code-blue situations don't survive—these kits might help. I asked her if she would be kind enough to get the kit, and she did. It contained an Ambu breathing bag to help with ventilation and a computerized defibrillator.

An Ambu bag requires a certain expertise to use effectively, and I happen to have that expertise while the security officer didn't, so I manned the Ambu bag and asked the security officer to pump on Patrick's chest, which she was able to do quite well. The defibrillator indicated ventricular fibrillation, which is the fatal heart rhythm just before flat line; defibrillation was unsuccessfully attempted, so pumping continued. After several minutes, Patrick's facial hue was just beginning to change from dark blue to light blue with a touch of pink around the forehead, which gave me hope.

Meanwhile, the code team was running over from the hospital, trying to negotiate the medical building and gathering numbers as they gathered momentum. By the time they arrived, they were twenty strong. They moved patients out of the waiting room and office except for a woman who was trapped in the other exam room at the end of the hall; she was unable to open the door to get out of the exam room because the place was jammed with medical equipment and personnel.

I have piles of paper forms, charts, computers, copiers, and fax machines in my tiny office, and everything nearby was rapidly shoved aside, causing papers and machinery to fly all over the place as resuscitation stuff was pushed into the office and exam room: intubation kits, IVs, oxygen tanks were strewn about, and my secretaries and medical assistants were huddled together, worried about Patrick, whom they were quite fond of, and weeping, while orders were shouted by the newly arrived code leaders. The scene was one of chaos, and the poor woman stuck in the back exam room would periodically squeeze the door open against a crush of bodies, peer out, and then slam the door shut. My office morphed, trashed like some wild frat party or one of those George Booth cartoons in the *New Yorker*. One of the waiting patients, a physics professor, kept looking at his watch and shouting to my secretary that his appointment was for fifteen minutes ago. Most of the patients who had been waiting simply looked dazed.

After twenty minutes of this and four more defibrillations, a pulse was noted. Patrick had a pulse! Soon he had a blood pressure and was immediately wheeled to the emergency room where he was bundled up and transferred via ambulance to Massachusetts General Hospital for urgent cardiac catheterization. He continued to remain unresponsive in a post–cardiac arrest hypoxemic coma. Via cardiac catheter, a metal stent was used to repair his totally occluded left anterior descending coronary artery ninety minutes after I first started pumping on his chest. He was cooled down in order to limit brain damage, which often results from low oxygen flow to the brain during cardiac arrest, and kept on a ventilator.

Three days later, Patrick was sitting up in bed in the coronary care unit at MGH, reading the newspaper. Three weeks after that, he was home, completing the *New York Times* crossword puzzle, worrying about the economy, and complaining about the bitter New England cold.

As an intern, I was expected to attend cardiac arrests that occurred in the hospital in order to learn how to save lives when the situation demanded, as it surely would—someday I would be in charge of cardiac resuscitation. On one particular occasion, a cardiac arrest (code blue) was called for a young girl with a previously undiagnosed heart problem as the result of a prolonged QT interval. She was at the hospital for a routine visit in order to follow up on her problem and to determine the effect of treatment for periodic seizures. As it turned out, she began to suffer from one of these seizures in the hospital office area. Typically, when her symptoms occurred, she would fall and her body would shake for several minutes. Then she would then relax and awaken. But during this particular event, she did not awaken and her pulse and blood pressure were unobtainable. The diagnosis had been wrong. We later learned the seizures were due to low oxygen supply to her brain as a result of a serious cardiac arrhythmia. She was resuscitated and ultimately required the placement of an implantable cardiac defibrillator. I never made it to the cardiac arrest. In my haste to get to her, I twisted my left knee (the same knee that kept me out of Vietnam), and I underwent knee surgery the next day. But I learned something about arrhythmias and about not accepting easy answers. A few years later, that young girl became my patient, and due to a weird twist in our health-care system, I fought to get her certain treatments rejected by her insurer. I succeeded then but would fail today because the insurance networks have increased the number of detours in the path to proper medical care.

For years, medicine in America was without equal and its doctors were devoted. As technology improved, patients lived longer and survived illnesses that used to kill or maim them.

The costs rose primarily due to the increased cost of advanced technology. In an attempt to reduce costs, systems were devised. Administrators were added in bulk to manage the systems.

As restrictions were placed on doctors, saving money (not lives) became the norm. We are told computer documentation is crucial and that we will be held responsible for rising costs. The fact is that insurers determine payments regardless of what the doctor chooses to charge. It is the rare physician who profits by recommending a test or treatment. What they feel is important for their patient is no longer of value to anyone except the patient and the doctor. We are told health care, once outstanding, was actually awful and the new changes create great care, but in truth, they create great profits for hospital, insurance networks, as well as the computer systems, which are redundant and create inefficiencies. Although claiming to exist only for the benefit of the ill, it is a profit-centered business.

It is in all our interests to have a system in which the doctor is empathetic and takes primary responsibility for patient care. They receive this mantle that has been passed through generations like a special chocolate recipe handed to a great-great-grandchild from a family of chocolatiers.

I write this in order to encourage young doctors to keep listening and for patients to realize that they need to be heard.

MEDICINE:
MANY YEARS BEFORE THE SAVE

In 1984 Libby Zion, an eighteen-year-old Bennington College student, presented to New York Hospital emergency room with vague symptoms thought to be of viral nature. She had been taking antidepressant medication. As part of her care, the intern and resident chose to give her pain medication to treat her symptoms. An unusual drug interaction occurred, resulting in her death. At that time, most doctors were unaware of this interaction. Libby's father, Sydney Zion, was understandably distraught. He was an influential attorney and had been a well-known newspaper columnist. He was able to parlay his anger into a high-profile case, resulting in the reduction in training hours for interns and residents.

Long before the Libby Zion laws reduced the hours doctors-in-training spent following their sickest patients in the hospital, we medical students trained with nervous, twitching eyes aimed toward the most experienced physicians while wondering what was going on in those remarkable medical minds. It was during that time that I began to cover the clinics as an anxious medical student. I believed I had contracted each disease I studied, especially the fatal ones. The fear hung over me like a death cloud. For example, I studied an insidious outbreak of brain worms (cerebral cysticercosis) in an unsuspecting group of vacationers soaking up sun in Jamaica. This particular disease was the result of soaking up much more than sun. It was acquired by ingesting salad that was tainted when the lettuce was washed with water contaminated by an infestation of pig tapeworm (*Taenia solium*) eggs. The allegedly clean water used to soak the lettuce had been sullied by deposits of worm-containing pig feces (the sanitation standards weren't quite up to snuff).

If one ingests the eggs, they can hatch, migrate through the intestines, travel through the bloodstream, and lodge in various organs as little tiny worms; they'll grow bigger and bigger until they finally cause symptoms. Cerebral cysticercosis means that the organ site that the worm visits is the brain; there, those wiggling, mischievous worms establish a residence and inhabit the brains of unlucky victims who have ingested the egg. When I first heard about this, I thought, *That can happen?* And then, because medical students often think they've contracted the gruesome diseases they study, I had it. After all, I had the occasional peculiar headache, and I too had eaten lettuce (albeit in Michigan, not Jamaica, but close enough).

Having survived my imagined illness, I can now tell you there are some things that take getting used to, like recurrent episodes of frightful diseases, and some things that you never seem to comprehend, like the nature of human response. It is a dizzying notion, and frequently it took getting it wrong, making an erroneous judgment, until finally getting it right—to suffer at first, then to master what I had not previously known. We may be quite certain, but we are also allowed to accept uncertainty as part of what makes for medical acumen and is the underpinning of our expertise.

And so for a while I trundled along, as if in the throes of death, fearing that I would soon expire from each one of the diseases I studied. I thought of myself as remarkably courageous when I would casually mention to nonmedical friends the fact how I was facing this or that fatal disease and was still soldiering on. "Tell no one, no need for pity here," I often said. But as time went by and I was still alive, I concluded, with a mixture of surprise and relief, that I must not have had that particular mortal illness after all. Thus, eyes open, breathing, with a pulse and a somewhat functional mind, I was able to move on to the next level of medical education.

I finished medical school and became a doctor, but all that really meant I was just a medical student with an MD after my name. So much of my education was ahead of me. Suddenly I was an intern and was expected to know what I was doing. Every patient has a medical problem that needs to be diagnosed and treated, and doctors at this level are expected to know the answers, to save lives. The sense of responsibility is daunting. One does what one can, afraid to make mistakes, but of course, making mistakes is impossible to avoid.

It was then that I met Peter S. He was about my age and, so like me, had his whole future ahead of him. Except he didn't. He had metastatic testicular cancer. His oncologist informed me that there was nothing more that could be done and Peter had come to the hospital to die. In those days, the treatment options were limited, and it seemed to me that the life of an oncologist must be quite depressing and awful. I also resented the fact that he gave up. I was young, and to my mind, medicine was not nuanced. I didn't think doctors were supposed to give up.

Over the next few days, Peter had trouble breathing, and treatments were only temporizing the inevitable as he spiraled downward. The night I thought he would die, I sat with him. He told me he was scared, so I held his hand and stayed with him, expecting his last gasp to occur at any moment. Eventually, I fell asleep, and in the morning, his parents walked in and found me sound asleep, holding Peter's hand. He was still alive. I was embarrassed to be found sleeping and excused myself, mumbling something about having just dozed off. They said nothing. Peter died two days later with his parents by his side. Shortly thereafter, Peter's cousin paged me to ask if I would be a pallbearer at Peter's funeral. A few years later, when I went into practice, Peter's parents were among my first patients.

But that is not the point of the story. I was an intern and was permitted to do whatever I felt was right, humane, and necessary. Perhaps what I did was helpful to Peter and his family, but it was equally meaningful for me—that's why I remember it more than thirty years later. It was a lesson in compassion that didn't really seem significant at that time. Many of my peers have similar stories, yet today new interns will never have these stories. They can't. Ever since the Libby Zion laws, training hours have been reduced in order not to overwork interns and residents.

That goal sounds eminently sensible. But years ago, it was considered irresponsible to abandon a critically ill patient, sign them out to another doctor, and leave simply because your shift has ended. The new rules limiting hours will result in a reprimand of the resident who stays late as well as a potential loss of accreditation for the training program that violates the rule. If the resident stays past his or her shift in spite of how important they feel it is to remain, they will be criticized.

The law claims to reduce medical errors, but this has not been proven. Yet with increased numbers of "hand-offs," the errors multiply like the misinterpretations in the game telephone. No intern, resident, or hospital is anxious to document errors as a result of following the mandated limits, so those errors are often ignored. We have been forced to follow a regulation with poorly documented benefits. Fewer hours are supposed to reduce risk and reduce errors; as I think back, I'm unconvinced. A medical student will graduate in June and start an internship in July. The time interns need in July and August in order to learn new things and to care for patients is much different than the amount of time they need in June after a year of training and experience. Spending longer hours allows for more experience, which is critical during those early months of internship. They may think of a diagnosis and perform a treatment without witnessing the result of their intervention because they are forced to abandon the patient to the next shift in order to comply with regulations. Strictly limiting hours while mandating both computer data entry and meetings with case managers to ensure rapid patient discharge cuts into both learning and patient care. I worry that allowing a sense of compassion and responsibility to be trumped by an inflexible rule carries great risk. I think Peter's family would agree.

As training continued with its massive piles of medical complexities, I met patient after patient, zeroing in on their diseases, but very little else (after all, these were relatively brief encounters focusing on the illness and only geared toward rapid diagnosis and treatment). They were all medical mysteries to be sorted out, and I generally bungled my way toward a resolution. Repetition made me more competent, and the formerly mysterious became clear as I gained more experience. I learned a diagnosis comes at you in a variety of ways; it can strike your senses. With repeated exposure, you can figure out what's happening by smell, sound, or feel, like the smell of newly mowed grass that elicits a memory recalling only one thing: cut grass. You can walk down a hospital corridor and know that there is a GI bleeder (blood pouring into the stomach or intestine) by its peculiar foul odor; the sound of whistling stridor associated with upper-airway disease is noticeable from the patient's doorway; the painless rock-hard mass on a patient's body tells your fingers they are touching a cancer. For doctors, these sensory experiences unlock mysteries. With the experience and knowledge I gained, I became more efficient at figuring out what was ailing my patients, and this allowed me to spend extra time talking with them. I could begin to gather extra tidbits about the patient's life; people open up when you're trying to help them.

This took a while, because during those intense early years, I didn't quite get it. While working in the hospital, I noticed how tight the rapport was between the older "gray beard" doctors and their patients. Initially, I found it odd that those doctors didn't spend as much time getting to know the patient's problem (while I spent lots of time and still made glaring errors) until I realized that the doctor knew so much about the patient that it was like having a family member with an extraordinary degree of medical knowledge. They knew their patients. I mean, they really knew their patients like a mother hen knows its chicks. This doesn't happen so much anymore, but it was quite common back then. (That is, before the advent of managed care and the overwhelming influence of bureaucratic health-care administrators.) Doctors were both confident and satisfied with the knowledge that they had about the person they were treating, and they appreciated the fact that they were the special recipients of trust.

It was a revelation when I realized that the old, wizened patient was not a chore to be dealt with as I sorted out the "medical mystery" of their illness. Instead they were a source of history and inspiration. This was getting to be not only medically challenging but also agreeable as I began to relish those encounters for more than just the medical evaluation. I was grateful for the opportunity for intellectual growth in addition to the degree of accompanying compassion that evolved from those unique interactions. The author and surgeon Dr. Richard Selzer referred to this experience as "mortal lessons," and as you will see, these stories provide just that—mortal lessons. It turns out that this connection with patients becomes a powerful weapon when fighting against the onslaught of the insurance network, which has lately been working in defiance of our better instincts. It doesn't hurt to advocate for your patient from a position of knowledge and empathy, to feel that you have a proprietary interest in the well-being of your patient. After all, it is your job, and it is the right thing to do.

The days of fearing that I would succumb to each new disease I came in contact with are long past, and I now see each patient not as a disease but as a source for understanding and gaining knowledge of society. With each story, I wondered how my patients survived or even triumphed. How did they make it through their ordeals? By virtue of listening to their stories, I continue to develop empathy and sensibility as they describe their descent, their ascent, and their survival. I attempt to stick by them. The stories from patients do not serve to shock; they are not meant to, but they do astonish. At the very least, they may be considered cautionary tales. Like most practicing physicians, I have been privy to a multitude of patient stories, which create images of the past and serve to reveal as they weave and intertwine through memory banks of the people who repeat them. It's best to listen while you can. We are an aging population, and the fact is that it will be crucial to develop compassion and interest in the elderly in order to progress as a society.

I once was going over a case with a medical student. It involved an elderly man suffering from vascular disease plus heart and lung failure, which is a fascinating problem for students. I understood that as a collection of symptoms, it was medically interesting to the student, but I worried that his interest in the patient as a person was limited. I should add that it was the same for me when I was a student—there's only so much energy we think we can exert per patient. In response to economic pressures inherent in our bizarre health-care system, the patient was being rushed through the hospitalization and readied for discharge to a nursing home. The elderly are especially exposed to the risks of a system that will rapidly push the patient to low-cost care: palliative care. If you are too old or too sick, it can be costly, yet with appropriate care, it is possible to prolong life. The issue is whether function and quality of life can or even should be maintained. Frustrated with the emphasis on moving patients out before they are adequately stabilized, I decided to teach the student a little bit more about the patient, to expose him to something new, and to add a bit of background in order to "humanize" the encounter and possibly gain more hospital time, something I felt was needed for a shot at further recovery. When teaching, it helps to remember that the best part of education is the surprise that comes from learning something you don't know that you don't know.

The patient was quite frail, in his eighties. He wore thick glasses and squinted, which caused his narrow face to crinkle into a smile. He was charmingly inquisitive, consistent with his life as a successful engineer; in fact, he had been instrumental in developing the "hotline," which was our coded emergency communication system with the USSR during the Cold War. It was a time when we were afraid that the United States and the Soviet Union were on the brink of a nuclear catastrophe and could, conceivably, blow each other up in a nuclear conflagration. This coded communication system was in place to prevent escalation of hostilities and, hopefully, to prevent nuclear war. It is common wisdom that the nuclear scenario ensures mutual destruction. Indeed, the hotline was utilized by the leaders of the United States and Russia (Kennedy and Khrushchev) during the Cuban missile crisis in the 1960s. During those early years, our patient had been appointed by the United States Army as a colonel (one of the few civilians to be so named); he was considered a national treasure (I didn't know that we had people who were named as national treasures, and by his admission, I discovered that he was one of a handful, which meant military battalions would be alerted wherever he traveled). His knowledge was highly classified and extremely important to our national defense. Our ill, dyspneic, half-blind elderly patient might have once saved the world.

I took the medical student to the patient's bedside in order for him to hear the story in the patient's own words, taking time to tell it between wheezes, as he struggled to breathe and speak at the same time. "I first [gasp] studied [wheeze] engineering [cough] at Yale... In the 1970s, NORAD [North American Aerospace Defense Command] thought that our early-warning radar system detected a Russian missile attack and initiated a response, which would have destroyed most of the world. A Canadian colonel was the only one who refused to accept the radar report and canceled our attack. He was right, and my team was brought in to figure out what happened. By using Doppler pulses, similar to those you used on my legs to check blood flow, we were able to determine what caused the misinformation. A rare event had occurred whereby the moon, sun, tides, and reflective surface of the earth created pulse oscillations [called the 17th reparate] that mimicked a missile attack. We identified and fixed the problem so that we no longer make that mistake."

He went on to describe his role in the 1960s with the hotline and the Cuban missile crisis. My student stepped back wide-eyed, and I hoped he would now consider spending extra time getting to know his patients. Maybe, just maybe, others had a story to tell.

The next day on rounds, I overheard him relating the story of the patient to other members of the house staff. I would like to believe that this contributed to the decision that was made to keep the patient in the hospital for a few extra days so that he could receive pulmonary rehabilitation before returning home with nursing services. It was a small triumph. I would hope it serves as a model for others. The elderly patient's story had a direct effect on at least one patient and one prospective doctor.

There remain millions of these interactions out there. It would be nice to affect a few more. Like other professions, medicine has a top-down learning process where medical students learn from interns and residents who learn from fellows and practicing physicians; responsibility must be taught in that manner.

As medical students we are innocent, wide-eyed enthusiasts until we, as interns and residents, learn to be skeptical, which gives way to cynicism. Then, with time and experience, if you live long enough, wisdom circles back around to innocence, enthusiasm, and a belief in the value of humanity. I've seen this happen. As the Fool said in Shakespeare's *King Lear*, "Thou shouldst not have been old till thou hadst been wise."

In this book, I have included patients' stories. With their permission, I tape-recorded and transcribed their accounts of their lives. Often, the telling of the story was cathartic for the patient, and on occasion, it appeared that healing came from that catharsis. In the case of Michael W., as his story unfolded, he noted a resultant release from pain, with lessening of chest pressure, maybe due to a change in stress hormones such as catecholamines (adrenaline), or perhaps the sense of relief is due to some other factor we have yet to uncover. Whatever the reason, I often find that dredging for and bringing out the stories helps patients. It certainly helps the doctor to know the patient better, and that can't hurt.

Many of these stories involve traumatic events, and some are so shocking that I am unable to respond in any comforting or comfortable manner, as in the case with the Nazi collaborator Petros. I can't tell if unearthing his tale helped either of us, but he definitely wanted to tell it. Perhaps he expected me to forgive him. As shocking as some of the stories are, each anecdote, each patient becomes part of the intricate tapestry that creates understanding and, perhaps, compassion. Or just the simple empathy found in those caged rats. Just like with the medical students who think they have each disease they study, a new world of experience evolves with each interaction.

Empathy developed surreptitiously as I found myself asking, "How am I similar to this person? How do I differ?" As the stories unfolded, the responses changed and evolved. With each attempt to answer these questions, we, physicians and patients (and everyone for that matter), learn something about ourselves. Without an appreciation of the life story of a patient, the medical student easily falls into the trap of viewing patients with a degree of detachment and cynicism. This attitude is all too frequent in our medical system these days, with all too many doctors and insurance-driven "case managers" acting as though patient care is a chore. To them, care is not about the person from whom we learn and whom we are called upon to heal. Among young doctors, this seeming callousness is often a protective bluff employed to cover inexperience. It is with experience, humility, and time that physicians evolve beyond the shell of cynicism while continuing to look both forward to bioengineering and backward to the lessons of Hippocrates in order to form the chimeral features of modern medicine.

The ancient Greek author Aeschylus wrote the Oresteian trilogy (the story of a cursed family) in order to instruct his audience about how to behave and to teach a degree of moral justice during this particular era. He concluded that civilization needs a few guidelines, such as don't kill kindred and don't behave treacherously to a guest or a host. Dante reserved treachery for the ninth circle of hell. Similarly, Eastern and Western religions incorporate stories to develop both a narrative and a belief system to teach a moral or ethic, ordained by a set of regulations: don't steal, kill, covet, and that sort of thing—you must have heard it somewhere. They determine how everyday issues are to be addressed based upon a philosophical and historical foundation.

These allegorical stories help us set our compass to figure out the direction we hope to take in our lives. Conveniently, this holds true for contemporary stories (our stories), because we will often use them as a mirror to reflect back on society. The story may lead to immediate change of direction, or it may seep in and cause a shift as imperceptible as that of the movement of tectonic plates. By the end, we should, at least, not kill kindred and not behave treacherously: do unto others.

Stories serve to remind us that it is part of our personal development to be at a crossroads whereby life takes a turn and changes as part of our developmental process. You never know when the change will occur. It's an old concept that change occurs by subtle twists, like that described in 460 BCE by the Greek philosopher Democritus that swerving tiny particles called atomi create everything from rocks to animals. Alternatively, momentous change was reported from the biblical writings in Genesis. We are taught to expect certain revelations: sudden light, then a serpent reveals the secret of mortality, for it was mortality, not nakedness, that delivered us from the Garden of Eden. It is butting up against mortality that results in the deepest of changes.

Change and bad news can be quite rapid, but for most of us, the change is the result of something mundane, barely noticeable, part of the continuum, just like a moment of any day. Is it that first time you fully understood birth, or is it the first time you hold the hand of a dying ninety-year-old woman? It doesn't matter when that moment is, but you start counting from then, looking forward, permitting you to overcome despair in order to cling to hope and, possibly, to develop wisdom.

THE FIRST TIME

From dust . . . released from a several-billion-year-old supernova, the stuff of human beings is a jumble of electrons that come together, build upon positive and negative charges, and combine to make atoms of carbon, hydrogen, oxygen, and nitrogen. Purines and pyrimidines are created and bind to high-energy phosphate to form nucleic acids, then, in a wondrous twist, they make DNA and RNA, which create amino acids that result in the manufacture of protein, and all that makes us. It is straightforward, like an automobile assembly line, almost simple. All the elements are in place, and the process moves along in a well-ordered manner until the moment of birth. Yet all births are not the same; if you have seen one, you have not seen them all.

    The first time I saw a birth was as a third-year medical student. I was taken in to observe. Standing in the back of the delivery room, behind the obstetrician, I was facing the action but not close enough to be of any assistance. I edged closer within this large windowless room that smelled of antisepsis and cleaning solutions. The mother was a seventeen-year-old black girl, her feet up in the stirrups, her pregnant belly swaying as she screamed, heaving and writhing throughout the pushing and the delivery. This was her third child, each with a different father. Her boyfriend, a tall, muscular black man in T-shirt and jeans, stood next to me. I had the sense that he viewed me as an intruder, and I guess, that's what I was. I found her shrieks of childbirth pain upsetting and was unnerved by the pervasive sense of chaos. It appeared to me that the orifice in question was too small for the task at hand, and I wanted to mention to the medical team that there must have been a gross miscalculation. Didn't anyone else notice?

The nurses acted rapidly and in what seemed to me a haphazard manner, as they moved about in response to commands made by the seated obstetrician, a plump, brusque middle-aged white man with an ample behind. I had assumed childbirth would be a wonderful, serene event. In spite of the drab Detroit day, I had imagined a contented mother, a supportive father, and a cooing baby, under blue skies filled with ballooning clouds floating joyfully in the atmosphere. This mother was not having any fun. Nor was her boyfriend, who grimaced with each scream and periodically looked at me menacingly (hey, it wasn't my fault). Deep within the recesses of my mind, as a way to keep myself from overt panic, I reviewed my textbook knowledge of childbirth and thought about the various forceps and cesarean deliveries I had studied. Although I tried to be cool, I was beginning to perspire in response to the moment and the warm August day (air conditioning was a rarity in inner-city Detroit). I heard the nurse ask, "How are you doing?" I started to answer that I was holding up fairly well, but before I could speak, I realized that she was addressing the patient, not me, and I was both embarrassed and further distressed. This was not the beautiful scene I had envisioned, and I wanted to raise the notion of major anesthesia for either the mother or, perhaps, for me. Where was the joy? Why would any thinking human being ever go through this ordeal?

Then, the baby started to crown; its scalp covered by wet hair started to show, then, startlingly, and it seemed to me unexpectedly, out popped the baby's head and some blood, then the rest of the tiny new life, a wiggling baby. It was letting out its first cry, and I was beaming and wanting to hug the smiling boyfriend, who was probably wondering who the giddy asshole standing next to him was.

The poet William Wordsworth once wrote that he was "surprised by joy." In this moment of unexpected joy, I realized how lucky I was to be in this situation, to be in medical school, and to be learning to be a doctor. I had just witnessed something miraculous; birth is a manifestation of how hope defies logic—a birth, a clue to the future. Maybe I will do this for the rest of my life!

That theme constantly reemerges in medicine. There are a myriad of medical problems that a person can encounter and overcome over the course of a lifetime. Even at a birth, questions arise. In this case, the question was glaring: what is the future for this newborn at risk? Yet I, along with his parents, could only hope . . . maybe this one would defy the statistics. The birth, like air bubbles in water slowly rising ultimately make it to the top, each ascending at their ordained speed, until finally one hits the surface and pops open to infinite possibilities.

From birth to death, there remains that constant attempt to find safety, happiness, a degree of success, and meaning; there is, indeed, with generosity and luck, a chance that each individual will achieve a full measure of his or her possibilities. But as the patients' stories attest, life is filled with roadblocks, some trivial, some tragic. Is this just one big Ponzi scheme, with each person's failure some other person's success? What keeps them going? For crying out loud, why don't they quit? It's a struggle seasoned by time, and simply making it to the surface is not enough. Somehow, in spite of adversity, we push on, hoping that the next roadblock will be the last.

I am reminded of a scene from a John Cleese movie where the hero keeps getting diverted from his destination by a series of humorous yet unfortunate events. Just as he is about to reach his goal, another problem arises and he has to start over. At one point, he is so disappointed that he sits on a curb at the side of a road, with his head in his hands, and he mumbles, "It's not the despair, I can handle despair . . . it's the hope."

My experience during medical training and throughout my career in medicine contains examples of both despair and hope, yet in my attic apartment that night after I first witnessed a birth, I only experienced hope. As I write this, I wonder, thirty-five years later, what happened to that wiggling baby boy born on a scalding August day. Then again, the mother, father, and baby have no idea what happened to me. In the end, medical education has provided a context of meaning as basic science gives way to notes on the human condition and then how it passes . . . to dust.

The major trauma hospitals in those days were located in places like New Orleans, the south side of Chicago, the Bronx, and the trauma center of them all: Detroit. Like today, things weren't so great for people living in Detroit. Those of us with experience working in those areas can tell the same stories as the people working in them today. On the occasions when we do gather to talk, we all find it astonishing that the situation has continued to fester without abatement over several decades.

PERCENT

My third-year medical school rotation found me stationed in the surgical emergency room at Detroit General Hospital as part of basic surgical trauma training. In 1974, Detroit was 70 percent black and 30 percent unemployed. The city is like a wheel with Detroit Center the worn-out hub shooting rusted spokes out to the periphery. Boarded-up and burned-out homes lined these roads that extended out to the 100 percent wealthy white circles on the periphery, where money was made by the auto industry. Violence and trauma in Detroit were as common as cocktail parties in the surrounding suburbs; I never saw the cocktail parties, but witnessing trauma was another thing.

Screaming ambulances arrived at Detroit General Hospital with striking regularity. One afternoon, a thing young bloody black male arrived at the emergency room with a shotgun blast to his chest and abdomen. Sixty percent of his intestines were blown away. The surgeons rushed him to the operating room and began an eight-hour repair (as I, the junior member of the team, held retractors to allow better views of the surgical site). Remarkably, they sutured various parts together, using a then novel procedure to attach the esophagus to the last part of the small bowel. (This turned out to be a poor plan, but who knew?)

The air we breathe is 21 percent oxygen, and normally that will saturate about 95 percent of our blood. But in trauma cases, such as the shotgun-blast recipient, fluid shifts occur, the oxygen doesn't get through the lung tissues as easily, and it is difficult to provide an adequate percentage of oxygen to the tissues; his oxygen saturation was about 75 percent. Thus, we gave him extra oxygen, and he survived to the point that he was able to converse and move about on his bed in the intensive care unit. But he was not to move from his bed for a couple of reasons: medically, it was unsafe, and he had killed a man. Therefore, the police had handcuffed him to the bed in order to prevent escape. My job was to monitor his vital signs and fluid input and output and to report to the intern (whom I thought knew everything). Unfortunately, as the patient became stronger, he became more belligerent and insisted that he be given something to drink. I advised him that the sutured intestines would break down and leak into his belly if he even sipped half a glass of water. IVs were providing liquid and nutrition to him; he didn't need to drink. He found me annoying. He explained to me where he thought I came from, who I was, and even where I could go. It was a most unpleasant conversation.

At the Detroit General Hospital in those days, the intensive care unit was one enormous room with bedridden patients attached to lifesaving equipment. They were lined up next to each other around the walls with the nurse's station in the center. The unit was understaffed, and everyone was overworked. In one corner of the room stood a refrigerator, which held enormous cans of juice so that the staff could keep well hydrated during work. Occasionally, a staff member would leave to eat or to use the bathroom, and that person would try to make sure someone remained to watch the patients. Due to the understaffing, however, this wasn't always possible. I was in the emergency room, and no one was staffing the ICU when the handcuffed patient swung his leg over the bed, dragged himself (bed and all) to the refrigerator, and downed most of a gallon of grapefruit juice. This prolonged his hospitalization, and it took several weeks to get him well enough to go to spend the next few decades in prison.

The trauma teams take all comers, caring for those from all walks of life, regardless of economic status or insurer. They do this because they are dedicated and enthusiastic about their work. At the moment, there is grave concern that there are fewer cultural and economic incentives to train trauma specialists. This situation is compounded by declining desire to provide care in poorly reimbursed trauma cases, and thus, a lack of experienced trauma teams. The president and legislators, for reasons of personal safety, can choose to avoid visiting these areas of high trauma and limited care (just in case . . .), or they can provide leadership in order to expand medical coverage and training in those areas, which will remain high risk for trauma and violence for the foreseeable future. The financial incentives for practicing preventative, such as eating right and getting plenty of exercise, clearly miss a significant segment of our population.

You would think that life in the violent inner city would be front-page news because it felt like a war zone in our own country. Yet it was part of the backdrop, not truly worthy of investigative reporting. It's been kept deep within the recesses of our minds. We knew things were bad in hidden parts of our country, but it is too difficult to solve, or so it seems. When the degree of violence and despair is revealed, it's overwhelming.

MEDIA

It's been years since I shoplifted from a major chain. I first learned about shoplifting when I was living in the south side of Chicago and visited a neighborhood kid who lived in a decrepit walk-up. His mother sent us to the store to steal bread. I watched with the numbed, uninformed moral sense of the eight-year-old I was as my friend and his sister snatched the loaf. I thought it must be okay since a grown-up, a mother, sent us on this mission (in fact, I felt a little disappointed that my own mother wasn't sending me out in a similar manner). In those days, we had milk delivered to our steps, and the same neighbor children were sent out to steal our milk as well. My mother suspected the culprits, but I wouldn't break my vow of silence, and they weren't caught (maybe my mother knew, but was compassionate—we never really discussed it).

From other neighborhood kids I learned the art of shoplifting, although I got caught with a shirt tucked into my pants on my first attempt to get something from a nearby chain store. Getting caught didn't stop me; it just made me wary. Eventually, I went after records and food. When I became a hippie, I no longer viewed it as shoplifting, but as liberating the product from the oppressor. However, one time, the butcher in a supermarket caught me. Instead of notifying the police, he explained to me that he spent time cutting and packaging the meat, and my actions cost him and, ultimately, his family. The poor grocery clerk would have to explain the missing sirloin to the owners. He was both sincere and respectful toward me, and my shoplifting ended abruptly that day.

By the time I started medical school, my shoplifting days were a distant memory. I was in Detroit where the ravages of drug abuse, unemployment, and nonstop violence had taken hold. No one walked around the city at night unless well armed or well drugged. In the midst of this stood Detroit General Hospital, where the best trauma surgeons worked because the "best" trauma wound up there. I tried to spend as much time there as I could, seeing and doing as much as permitted (which was quite a lot). On occasional evenings, I would get a bite to eat and watch the evening news. The first fifteen minutes of the news were usually devoted to the murders of the day, and I felt a certain perverse pride knowing that, in some small way, I was part of those stories since I was often on emergency room duty when the murderer or the victim came in for urgent care. It was all new and exciting and did not bother me much until the day that a middle-aged black female shoplifter came in dead on arrival, or DOA. Identified as Jane Doe, she was the single mother of two. The police had shot her in the back of the head as she was running away—she had stolen two pounds of ground beef from the local grocery chain. I noticed the meat jammed in her jacket as she lay dead on the gurney.

That evening, I was glued to the TV, awaiting her story on the news. The following day, I combed the papers for the report. It was never mentioned.

Sometimes, sifting through rocks in a vacant lot, the neighborhood kids and I would turn a large rock over and find a community of insects scattering as it was exposed to the sun. Some of us found it disgusting, but for others of us, it was fascinating. When Hurricane Katrina broke through the levees and revealed the underbelly of society, the reaction was similar. This did not surprise those of us who had experience with the inner city where neglect runs rampant and sympathy is hard to find. The rock eventually gets turned back over, and we move on, never thinking about what damage we might have inflicted on a community. The trauma physicians in Detroit remain there to repair what damage they can fix.

THE URINAL

"Doc, I gotta pee." My patient's stale, wine-soaked breath emitted a nauseating aroma as he pleaded to use a urinal. His huge facial gash had been cleansed, and I was in the process of placing several sutures above his right eye; a sterile drape covered most of his face. I would have completed the task and let him urinate, but my attention was diverted by sudden activity in the trauma room of the Detroit General Hospital emergency room where I was training in my third year of medical school. Still in the thrall of youth, each new case was fresh and exciting. I relished the new experiences and opportunities to learn.

Some people can't stand the sight of blood, but trauma surgeons at Detroit General are attracted to it like sharks at a feeding frenzy; the case, which diverted my attention, was one of those situations. The patient was bleeding from his neck, chest, and abdomen as a result of gunshot wounds. I was called over to help but tried to explain that I was busy and should probably be somewhere else. Before I could finish my excuses, the trauma team had staunched the bleeding in the neck and opened the chest, where they found a bullet hole in the heart. They proceeded to repair it and needed me to pump intravenous fluids into the patient. As they were barking orders, blood was spurting, and I tried to explain how ill-equipped I was for this sort of work. They had opened the abdominal wall and found that the abdominal aorta—the major artery leading from the heart to the lower half of the body—had been punctured by a bullet. Blood, bright red, arterial, was swirling and rushing forth. Thus began a voyage into the abdomen, which was a sea of blood with a sky of blue surgical masks above. They needed someone to apply pressure to the vessel in order to decrease further blood loss. Since I was already wearing sterile gloves, I was appointed the task of reaching into the ocean of blood, my hands and arms sailing deep into the abdominal cavity and finding and pressing down on the aorta. (These were pre-AIDS days, and no protection further than gloves was deemed necessary with severe trauma cases—although I noticed that the surgeons wore gloves, masks, and gowns.)

The patient managed to survive long enough to be wheeled up to the operating room where further repairs would be made. As we were transporting him out of the trauma room, I looked back to see my abandoned facial-laceration patient standing, suture and needle hanging from above his right eye, sterile drapes still covering part of his face, pants down and no longer able to wait, using the wall of the trauma room as a urinal.

There is something thrilling in new experience no matter how grotesque. It is fresh, enhanced by the innocence of youth. Joseph Conrad once wrote of old men sitting around near a dock, watching the great sailing ships come in, and discussing a young sailor's return from the sea: "By all that's wonderful it is the sea, I believe, the sea itself—or is it youth alone? Who can tell? But you here — you all had something out of life: money, love — whatever one gets on shore — and tell me, wasn't that the best time, that time when we were young at sea; young and had nothing . . . and we all nodded at him: the man of finance, the man of accounts, the man of law, we all nodded at him over the polished table that like a still sheet of brown water reflected our faces, lined, wrinkled; our faces marked by toil, by deceptions, by success, by love; our weary eyes looking still, looking always, looking anxiously for something out of life, that while it is expected is already gone - has passed unseen, in a sigh, in a flash - together with the youth, with the strength, with the romance of illusions."

Youth was passing like illusions, medicine and patients filling my senses, adding substance to the blank spaces, and it was seeping into the marrow of my bones, confounding idealism, skepticism, cynicism, nihilism with their despair, and my hope.

After Detroit, I continued my medical training in Boston, which had the reputation of being the hub of medicine. I noted that the Boston training center captured a distinctly different patient population than inner-city Detroit. I spent a great deal of time working in the intensive care unit, interspersed with time in the emergency room. I was developing a particular interest in the critically ill.

I didn't expect to recapture the feeling of lawlessness and rampant violence, but I was surprised to find the common thread of self-inflicted wounds as well as the seeds of self-destruction. No matter where we live, we humans certainly have a gift for creative self-destruction. It's not as though we haven't been forewarned.

ALCOHOL

Millicent enjoyed a nightcap—a cocktail, she called it. Even without the cocktail party, the ball, the dressing gown, the band, the milling around of millionaires, she would imagine an extravagant or romantic occasion and enjoy her cocktail event. As she daydreamed, she poured gin into an enormous goblet and wandered the rooms of her Victorian suburban home. As forty years passed, the home became shabbier, and so did she. Her skin took the yellowed pallor of an old and faded wedding dress, her face lined by the ravages of cigarettes and troubled sleep. She used alcohol in a futile attempt to recapture the lost lightness of heart from before she was alone. No matter how much and how often she poured herself a drink, it never seemed to be enough. Her thought became disorganized yet pressured, like salmon swimming upstream in order to return to spawn and to die, the alcohol helping to suppress the pressure and the chaos within her mind.

Cocktail hour began to occur earlier and earlier. By the time I spoke with her, she confessed to me it was starting around 10:00 AM; she couldn't say when it ended. The years of drinking had taken their toll. The car got banged up and was left in the garage to rot. She stopped going out. She called for deliveries of groceries and gin but then ran out of funds for groceries, and her credit at the liquor store went dry. That's when she was forced to rummage through her home for an alcohol substitute, and that's when she came up with a container of antifreeze. Since the car couldn't use it, she figured she would. Not surprisingly, it made her ill, but she managed to dial 911 in time and was taken to the hospital as she slipped into a coma.

When I saw her at first, I couldn't get the story straight; no one knew what had happened, and there was no one but Millicent who knew the story of the toxic ingestion. We only knew that she arrived in a coma and might soon be dead. The emergency team immediately called the intensive care team because it was obvious that she required intensive care. We had to piece the story together as we figured out ways to keep Millicent alive. She was only fifty-eight, but she looked seventy-eight. The smeared red lipstick had been messily applied days before, probably around the time she last brushed her tangled puffs of white hair. She had not been prepared to go out this day.

She was unable to be aroused, was unresponsive to verbal or physical stimuli, and had crystalline particles in her urine (a clue to her critical illness). Through blood tests, we discovered she had a low serum pH, indicating severe buildup of acid in her system. Imagine pouring sulfuric acid on paper, watching it smoke and burn. Severe acid buildup in the body has awful effects, but they don't announce themselves just as noticeably as the image of sulfuric acid smoke rising from the surface of paper. So it requires special studies. Acid levels can build up for a variety of reasons, such as infection, trauma, shock, and toxins, and all of them are life-threatening. We needed to figure out the cause as quickly as possible because Millicent's survival depended on correct treatment.

A clue to the cause of acidosis is found by measuring negative particles called anions. First, we had to figure out the amount of anions in her blood. Anions reveal the degree of negative charges in the body. Millicent had too many anions in her bloodstream causing the blood to be quite acidic. There was evidence of a rambunctious, presumably fatal, toxin attacking her body. The extent of the acid buildup can be determined by further studies of the blood.

It is understood that shifting fluid in the body occurs, in part, from shifts across cells and tissues in relation to osmotic loads created by chemicals. (These chemicals, which exist in the body, are part of a solution to allow water to either move away, toward, or remain in a cell, which is the basis of osmosis.) Dramatic shifts of these chemicals and fluids can lead to death, so it is important to check for osmotic fluid shifts when acid levels are high. The most important molecules involved in the shift are sugar (used for energy), salt (used for electrical activity), and urea (a by-product of protein metabolism). Once we knew the blood test values of those molecules, we could calculate the osmotic load and then compare that number with the osmols directly measured from a blood specimen. Normally, the calculation and the measurement of osmols are pretty much equal; if one value is significantly different from the other, as it was with Millicent, drastic action is needed.

We put Millicent on dialysis to compensate for failure of her kidneys, and we had to treat the underlying cause of Millicent's problem. Only a couple of toxins tend to cause this type of situation: methanol (long known by men who worked the illegal backwoods stills as a product of "wood alcohol" formed by distilling the vapors of heated wood), and ethylene glycol. Although the treatment is the same for both toxins, it helps to differentiate between the two in order to figure out how the toxin was obtained. From the crystals in her urine, we decided Millicent had ingested ethylene glycol (antifreeze). We had our answer.

The treatment for ethylene glycol toxicity requires inhibition of the enzyme alcohol dehydrogenase. This prevents production of toxic metabolites. Although now newer drugs (such as fomepizole) are available to inhibit alcohol dehydrogenase, we had only one such treatment twenty years ago. We needed to give her ethanol in order to compete with ethylene glycol for binding sites on the enzyme. In those days, you could pour high-proof booze (high percent in ethanol) in the dialysis bath, and it would get into the bloodstream and work its magic. It was effective; she survived, and when she finally aroused, she thanked us and was quite curious as to where we got the alcohol and asked if we had any left.

TURNING YELLOW

On occasion, people change colors with a chameleon-like turn of skin tone: red or brown might be indicative of sun exposure, yellow can indicate jaundice, and a blue tinge to the lips can be ominous. It is caused by lack of oxygenated hemoglobin, usually due to severe heart or lung difficulty. It can also result from a defect in hemoglobin's ability to carry oxygen, which is what happened to a group of men from the Bowery district in New York many years ago (as reported by the *New Yorker*'s great medical writer Berton Roueché). They didn't have lung or heart trouble—they were hungry and wanted to season their oatmeal. Unfortunately, they chose to use sodium nitrite instead of sodium chloride because it was such a cheap salt alternative. The trouble is that nitrite causes a change within the hemoglobin, which results in less oxygen affinity. When that occurs, you turn blue.

Occasionally, a doctor will choose a therapeutic modality that can cause the patient to turn blue. While working in the emergency room, I was confronted by a patient exposed to sudden cyanide release. Cyanide poisons the cell's power source (mitochondria), and if mitochondria fail, you die. When given an immediate inhalation of amyl nitrate, followed by injection of thiosulfate, converting to thiocyanate, a patient exposed to cyanide can survive because a molecule is formed, which will compete to bind cyanide, thus taking it away from the mitochondria.

The treatment creates the molecule methemoglobin, which will preferentially bind cyanide, thus protecting the mitochondria, but the cyanide now binds to the new molecule whereas oxygen can no longer bind tightly. The side effect is a brief resultant bluish skin tone. My patient received appropriate therapy and survived—blue in skin color only.

Hemoglobin plays a role in yellowing of patients as well. If red cells explode into pieces, the hemoglobin is released and breaks down to bilirubin, which is metabolized in the liver. If there is too much breakdown, the liver is overwhelmed and jaundice (yellow coloration) develops. The liver's role in bilirubin metabolism explains how liver disease can cause one to turn yellow; damaged liver cells no longer can metabolize bilirubin, so it passes through the liver and continues through the bloodstream. This may occur with viral illness resulting in viral hepatitis (from exposure to tainted food, water, needles, or bodily secretions). Alcohol toxicity can do the same thing. Abnormal copper metabolism as seen in young people with Wilson's disease is another cause. It occurs with infections such as those exposed to rat urine if it contains the bacteria *Leptospira*, mosquitoes with the protozoa causing malaria, and snails spreading the schistosoma parasite. That's not all. As bilirubin leaves the liver via the bile duct, its progress may be impeded by gallbladder disease or tumors resulting in reabsorption and, you guessed it, yellow skin color.

Years ago, Roger Z. came to see me with the complaint, "My friends think I look yellow and that I must have jaundice." He was in his thirties and quite a health nut. Although he was bright yellow, including the palms of his hands, the whites of his eyes showed no yellow. In true jaundice, the whites of the eyes turn yellow. However, I immediately knew the source of Roger's problem: he ate too many carrots. Carrots can cause the skin to turn yellow, including the palms, but sparing the white of the eyes. Roger confessed that he typically ate a dozen carrots daily. I advised him that that was his problem, and he asked, "What should I do with the bushels of carrots in my apartment?" I inquired if he had ever heard of the Bowery Bums. I didn't know if they were still around, but I assumed that someone in that neighborhood was hungry. In reply, Roger asked if garlic could cause color change.

Just as I was getting the hang of middle-class self-destructive behavior, something new would arise. I suppose this is analogous to what we all experience when we read the paper or hear the news and learn that another unexpected crisis has occurred. However, it is different when you are placed in the midst of the crisis, trying to gain perspective as you sort through the damage. While one patient is gravely ill, there is another immediately in danger and another after that. Often the nature of the case provides very little time to adjust and less time to sit back and assess the situation, which is, in part, why I write about it.

PHOSPHORUS

Susan E. came to my attention on the anniversary of Stendhal's birth. She frequently mentioned that he was her favorite author, and she carried a copy of his book *The Red and the Black* with her; it is a story of hypocrisy in France during the 1830s. You may know that the chemical carbon can create the color black, and manganese, the color red. However, though not mentioned by Stendhal, I find the more significant element to be phosphorus, in part because it can create light in the dark (I suppose that Stendhal tried to do that as well). We need phosphorus for more than light, but too much can cause problems. High doses of phosphorus can be toxic. Combined with certain chemicals, it forms pesticides that kill insects and get into the fat stores of fish and animals, causing damage to the nervous system. Ingesting white phosphorus causes smoking stool syndrome occurring when the phosphorus in the feces is exposed to air and warm clouds of white smoke rise up from the fecal load, and this billowing smoke indicates the presence of a toxic digestive tract filled with phosphorus. Yet to live in this world, we need phosphorus. When phosphorus is added to nucleic acids, it makes ATP (adenosine triphosphate), which is the fuel required by our cellular engines (the mitochondria).

Susan didn't like to eat. She had a severe case of anorexia nervosa, and she didn't seem to care. She had wasted away to sixty-seven pounds by the time I met her in the intensive care unit. Although she was about to slip into a coma, she had the unusual affect of a starving anorexic. She was weak, yet strangely euphoric, and said she felt fine. It was imperative to provide her with intravenous nutrients in order to keep her alive. As we replenished her sugar, she started to rouse. The sugar was necessary for metabolism in the cell via the Krebs cycle. As part of the process, phosphate was utilized to form more ATP to get the cellular engines going. As those mitochondria were humming away, they utilized more and more phosphate. The result of that was to lower the total body stores of phosphate to perilously low levels, and muscle cells broke down, releasing debris that clogged the kidneys. Susan's kidneys failed, and she required temporary dialysis. The nerves also needed phosphorus in order to function, and the nerves and muscles that aided breathing failed as she became paralyzed. We placed her on a ventilator machine in order to help her breathe.

She finally received enough phosphorus to get off the ventilator, and her kidneys and muscles gradually improved. She was up to eighty-eight pounds when she walked out of the hospital. I encouraged her to take in adequate nutrition, including milk, which is high in phosphorus. She was grinning while her eyes were seeking and furtive, until she passed a mirror in the hall. She looked puzzled and then concerned with the reflected image that she perceived. What she saw in her reflection was not what I saw when I looked at her and, especially, what I remembered about all we had gone through. She saw something different. Unfortunately, she felt she needed to go on a diet.

History doesn't repeat itself, but it does rhyme.

—Mark Twain

EXPECTATIONS

In 2011, the much-anticipated Hurricane Irene hit the Atlantic coast. Because of the heavy media coverage, people were prepared. They'd stockpiled bottled water, candles, flashlight batteries, and ice. They expected power outages relieved only by the flickering of flashlight-induced shadows on a wall reminiscent of Plato's cave (without the same philosophical interpretation, of course). Some hoped it would result in a time of quiet reflection, perhaps spent with friends and family in a cozy environment filled with the murmurs of pleasure as the happy, well-stocked group settles in to a simpler lifestyle.

For some, however, it brought about an itch. This is how Hurricane Irene struck Barbara H., whose daughter, three grandsons, their two dogs, and a cat settled in together for the duration of the hurricane. Barbara was prepared, or almost prepared. She was caught off-guard by one thing: a pruritic rash that she had developed a few days before she came to see me in the office. I informed Barbara, as I backed away from her, that the small clusters of itchy red bumps looked to me like flea bites. She said that she thought her daughter had rid the animals and kids of their flea problem, but clearly she was mistaken.

Fleas cause itchy rashes and, in notorious cases, carry serious disease. The bubonic plague of the sixth century, known as the Plague of Justinian, led to the decline of the Byzantine Empire (the eastern part of the Roman Empire). In the fourteenth century, the plague was called the Black Death, and it killed millions. In addition to the fear that this could be a sign from God, a major theory at that time was that Jews had poisoned the wells. In retribution, Jews throughout Europe were persecuted, attacked, and exterminated, including immolation of two thousand Jews in Strasbourg on St. Valentine's Day 1349. Winston Churchill once commented, "The further you look back in history, the better you can see the future."

As we now know, the poison theory was wrong. The plague was carried by fleas on rats that traveled with traders from China along the Silk Road. The disease that fleas carry is due to *Yersinia pestis*, a gram-negative coccobacillus named after the scientist Alexander Yersin. It was not poison that caused the plagues; it was a vicious bacteria passed on by fleas that traveled on rats.

Here's how they do it. It is thought that *Yersinia pestis* is mutated from *Yersinia pseudotuberculosis*, which can rest inside a flea's gut without causing a problem. But when *Yersinia pestis* gets into the gut of a flea, it's not harmless. It causes intestinal blockage that prevents the flea from digesting food. So now the starving, constipated, blood-devouring flea regurgitates its *Yersinia*-containing contents into the bloodstream of whomever it is feeding on—rat or human. If it's a rat, the rat blood simply serves as a reservoir for the bacterium, but in a human, *Yersinia pestis* can cause lymph nodes to swell and suppurate (causing what are called bubos, hence the name bubonic plague). It can be even more malicious, however, causing sepsis, pneumonia, disseminated intravascular coagulation, meningitis, and gangrene—hence the name Black Death.

As I scratched all over my body, I informed Barbara of the pressing need to eradicate fleas from her home and secretly hoped she could find another doctor if this reoccurred. But I harbored no special expectations.

BEAUTY

Walking down the fifth-floor corridor of the Boston area hospital I worked, I glanced into room 576, where I noticed a woman trying to crawl out of the window.

Several days earlier, I had cared for her in the intensive care unit. She had been admitted to the intensive care unit following a suicide attempt. She was an attractive middle-aged woman with dark-brown hair cut to shoulder-length, and she wore a modest amount of makeup on her full, expressionless face; one could imagine her tastefully attired. She had taken an overdose of belladonna.

Some say belladonna poisoning was the cause of the fall of the Roman Empire since it was a popular beauty aid during that era. Others say it was the lead in the water system and drinking vessels that weakened the populace. Edward Gibbon, the eighteenth century historian, wrote that it was the advent of Christianity plus the barbarian invasion that turned the tide and led to the decline of Rome and that belladonna wasn't really the culprit. But I think the idea of vanity leading to the destruction of an empire is both poignant and instructive. Irrespective of the cause of the fall, I'd stay away from belladonna. Belladonna is an atropine-like drug that has been known about even before the Roman Empire. This type of drug, called *laffa* by the Arabs and "mandrake" by the British, was once described as "love plant" because of the Old Testament belief that it improved the fertility of barren women. Atropine will affect the smooth muscles in the body, including those responsible for pupillary constriction. Women used small aliquots to dilate their pupils in order to become more alluring to men (belladonna, in Italian, means "beautiful woman"). This patient did not overdose in order to appear more beautiful (although beauty was on her mind). She was five and a half feet tall and weighed 170 pounds, and her husband preferred more slender women. He often told her how much he felt she had "let herself go."

An overdose of belladonna causes increased thirst, difficulty swallowing, headache, nausea, delirium, rapid pulse and respirations, excitement, hallucinations, and convulsions—it can be fatal. While in the intensive care unit, the patient's overdose was treated with the antidote physostigmine. Afterward, she was transferred to the fifth-floor medical unit for observation. On the day she decided to exit through the window, the psychiatrist, after conferring with the patient's husband, deemed her no longer suicidal and ready to return to the bosom of her family. She was to be discharged home. However, they were mistaken. The psychiatrist was filling out the usual discharge forms at the nursing station when I walked past. When I saw the woman at the window, I knew something about this scene didn't make sense, but it took me a couple of seconds to react, so I yelled, "Wait!" She didn't and continued to climb through the open window. I rushed in and grabbed for her hands and missed, but I was able to grab her right ankle and hold tight. She hung out the fifth-floor window, head down. She was dead weight, not putting up any resistance. It seemed quite weird to me. I mean, if you're attempting to kill yourself, why not struggle against the efforts of the rescuer? It wasn't until I reflected upon this that I realized that if you are so depressed that you are willing to kill yourself, it is possible that you are also too depressed to struggle—a true, overwhelming despair.

My knees had slammed into the radiator beneath the window, which was wide-open. I could hear the birds singing outside, perhaps urging me to hold on, perhaps mocking, and I felt a mild spring breeze blow into the room, creating a strange calmness to the world around us. Things felt like they were happening in slow motion, yet I know they weren't. I imagined losing my grip, resulting in her long fall, then the thud, her death, and my unrelenting guilt. I screamed for help. The staff initially thought that they were hearing the rants of the demented patient who shared the hospital room and did not respond with the urgency I felt the moment required; my knees were throbbing, and I was afraid I would let go. I yelled louder. Finally, after moments, which seemed like hours, a couple of nurses came in. One rushed out, and then a man from security arrived, and we pulled her back inside. The psychiatrist arrived on the scene and noted that maybe she should be transferred to a locked psychiatric ward. And she was. She didn't protest, expressing what French doctors have called *la belle indifférence* (the beautiful calm) seen in certain psychiatric cases.

Due to a quirk of fate, I had saved her life. Once, a few days later, I visited her on the psychiatric ward, expecting to be greeted as a conquering hero or given at least a modicum of gratitude. That was not to be. So after standing by her bedside for about five minutes, with little or no recognition of my deed, I left. I don't think she looked up as I said good-bye and walked out the door of her room on the psychiatric ward, expecting her to call out after me, perhaps with the word of thanks that never came.

However, I was commended by the vice president of the hospital and was told that I had saved the hospital from some awful publicity. The unctuous VP said that I should expect something beautiful from the institution. But I don't put much faith in beauty.

According to the *Iliad*, Paris discovered that Helen of Troy, the wife of Menelaus, was gorgeous. He seduced her and ran off with her to Troy. Menelaus and his brother, King Agamemnon, chased after them. Unfortunately, Agamemnon's ships were stuck in port because there wasn't enough wind for their sails. A prophet advised Agamemnon to sacrifice his daughter and the winds would come. The prophet was right, but he forgot to mention that when the war ended ten years later, Clytemnestra (Agamemnon's wife) wouldn't forget the death of their daughter. She murdered the king upon his return, another death in the service of beauty. The story was written in order to impart a moral and a message. It was expected that the reader would learn to be more careful, follow particular rules, and develop a few basic principles: don't be blinded by beauty, and don't harm your children. But religion of a different sort was taking hold in other parts of society, and those lessons have been ignored as exemplified in the following story.

LATENESS

Jimmy W. came in too late. He was twenty-one when I first met him and twenty-one when I last saw him. Because I had agreed to cover especially sick patients, I was assigned his case. He was very ill, but he didn't know it. All he knew was that his scrotum had swelled to the size of a cantaloupe, and he thought that was abnormal. He was right. Not only had his scrotum swelled, but his legs had swollen up to the size of those of a hippopotamus. The lower half of his body had filled with fluid because his heart, serving as a fluid pump, had failed to pump adequately. Gravity and elevated hydrostatic pressure had caused the fluid to gradually back up, starting with his feet and eventually creeping as high as his belly. But it was the scrotal swelling that alarmed Jimmy.

Jimmy was always a little different. As a child he was unable to keep up with the other kids; when running or playing sports, he would get easily winded. In addition, and poorly understood by Jimmy, he didn't grow nearly as tall as his brothers. Jimmy's family did not get too concerned. They were Christian Scientists, and when problems arose, they took him to the Christian Science healer who explained that Jimmy had asthma and could use a whopping dose of prayer.

It took a few years of prayer for Jimmy's scrotum to swell. Jimmy had been born with a hole in his inner heart wall, which separates different heart chambers. The heart wall has a protective mechanism that closes any of the problematic holes (formed normally as part of the fetal circulation, but correcting shortly after birth). As the baby matures, blood is prevented from being pushed in the wrong direction through the heart. Blood is pumped in a cycle through the body and replenishes itself with oxygen as it passes through the lungs. The hole in Jimmy's heart diverted the normal cycle flow and caused the heart to work harder. Over time, the heart developed an abnormal route, bypassing some of the life-sustaining oxygen in the lung. This put more pressure on the heart, and its muscular pump began to fail, causing the blood returning from distant parts of the body to back up and letting fluid leak from the swollen blood vessels into the surrounding tissues. It simply couldn't compensate for the lack of proper blood circulation. The result was a swollen lower body.

The hole in Jimmy's heart was the result of a birth defect, which is easily diagnosed and surgically treated in newborn babies or young children. I have seen many patients who are alive and well decades after this kind of heart surgery. Without the surgery, though, the heart fails and patients end up like Jimmy: short of breath, blue, with oxygen-starved lips and fingers, enormously swollen legs, and a huge fluid-filled scrotum. He gasped for breath with the slightest effort, and his eyes were large with fear, darting around, watching nervously as medical personnel came and went.

Jimmy was raised to be quiet and respectful. He expressed a concern that he was somehow responsible for his predicament. I sat with him as the intern and medical student tried to explain how this disease process was not his fault, but they could not allay his feelings of guilt and his certainty that he must be a sinner. Although he was twenty-one, he deferred to his parents and wanted them involved in all medical decisions. The diagnosis had been easily figured out and was explained to Jimmy and his mom and dad. The treatment required aggressive medical intervention, which would eventually include a heart and lung transplant. Although Jimmy's father was in agreement, his mother was concerned about the religious ramifications. She argued with the father until they decided it would be best to involve the healer from the Christian Science church before making a final decision.

I met with the healer and the parents for about an hour in my office—Jimmy was not present. The healer insisted that this was no time to leave the faith (this was a test that must be passed) and convinced Jimmy's mother that what was needed was more prayer. Jimmy's father, dealing with a process both grand and invisible, acquiesced again. I was frustrated and incensed as the healer smiled beatifically once the family reached their decision. I imagine that is the same satisfied smile of those who send suicide bombers to meet their fate.

They took Jimmy home and prayed and prayed, and the healer worked her magic. Jimmy died within two months.

Jimmy's family sold pianos, and I bought one from them after Jimmy's death. I don't know why. At that time, I was convinced that it was simply a matter of convenience; their piano store was nearby, and I would one day take piano lessons. The piano is now out of tune. I've not found the time or inclination to get it tuned properly; after all, I don't really know how to play, and . . . it's just a piano.

A LESSON

Since the time of Copernicus, the conflict between religion and science has raged, and it continues now in medicine, thanks to technological advances and the countervailing forces of religious zealots. In the second century, Galen tried to determine the effects of remedies, attempting to figure out how things worked, and wrote a thirty-volume pharmacopeia. He has been described as the last pharmacist for a millennium, supplanted by religious mysticism for the subsequent thousand years of the Middle Ages (also known as the Dark Ages) when treatments consisted only of "getting the demons out." What we now acknowledge as nonsense was accepted common practice—once upon a time. It took more than a thousand years to get back to scientific inquiry as an approach to disease. Doctors and laypeople alike are caught in the struggle to answer questions about quality of life, the beginning of life, and even how and when life should end. This is no longer the era of the Dark Ages—we should be more technologically sophisticated than our predecessors from those Middle Ages. However, medical science and religious belief are often at odds as questions are raised regarding end-of-life decisions and the sanctity of life. Physicians are often forced to make life-and-death decisions, influenced by religion and politics; we remain reliant on our experience—it's intrinsic to science.

For decades we have been swept up in the debate about abortion, and more recently, the question has been raised about what to do with tiny clusters of embryonic cells, which may be utilized as stem cells to help patients with devastating diseases. They may be used to correct spinal cord injuries, brain malfunctions, cancers, and heart damage. The stem cells are getting the attention that's richly deserved, but it comes at a price, both moral and political. There is an undeniable difference between a late-term fetus and that minuscule cell cluster. To get an idea of the size of the cluster, pick up a quarter and look at the profile of George Washington, then look at his nose and try to picture a hair on that nose; the cluster is smaller than that almost invisible hair. Those derive the stem cells.

When I was a medical student, it was not uncommon to assist with abortions, sometimes even taking a fetus (delivered with the help of an oxytocin-like stimulus) and taking it into a room where it could not be revived. Sometimes the abortions involved using implements to remove the fetus piece by piece with the segments quite identifiable: a hand, a torso, a leg. Abortion is an unsettling concept, but so are the consequences of not having abortions available. Often these were abortions for teenagers who had been raped or were victims of incest. During the days when it was difficult to find a doctor to perform an abortion, it was not unusual to find fifteen-year-old girls lying ill on the ward after an emergency hysterectomy performed to save them after a septic or hemorrhagic home abortion. Those were the survivors, that is, the girls who did not perish in the back room of their family homes after a botched abortion attempt.

It was also common knowledge that first-year college students would visit the clinic in the winter after having left home in late summer and, having made a mistake, wound up with an unwanted pregnancy, which would forever change their lives regardless of their choice. Some politicians and religious groups find themselves involved with what is clearly a difficult dilemma, but these groups bring so much dogma that it is impossible to have a reasoned dialogue. The issue is tough enough without antagonism between religion and science. Knowing science, developing compassion and experience, and listening to the patient help.

Regardless of the outcome, one remains strongly affected by the encounter and must rely on moment-to-moment decision making based upon those factors. We are forced to develop and be guided by a moral compass; for some it's established through laws, for others it's established by religious precepts, but I think, for most, it is experience and empathy that allow our opinions to form and to change. These stories provide a degree of experience, permitting us to develop and refine our personal moral and ethical standards.

Although not yet aware of societal and political changes in medicine, my frame of reference was expanding, and as it developed, my reactions became clarified, sometimes too late. I became more comfortable with my medical knowledge and gradually became aware of hints that there were stories beyond the illness, which at first was insidious, but eventually it took the jolt of my encounter with Rose A. ("Regret") to change focus. I renewed my attempt to listen and learn, trying to understand but not entirely reserving judgment. The patients have stories to tell, and they're best told, and listened to, before they are dead or demented. More often than not, the opportunity is squandered, and then it is too late.

REGRET

Rose, almost eighty years old, presented one night as I was working intensive-care duties. She was sent from a neighboring nursing home because she complained of chest pressure and air hunger—she was unable to catch her breath. With the standard tests (electrocardiogram and cardiac enzymes), we determined that she was suffering from a massive heart attack. I was among the first to care for her, and I was young and energetic. My idea of a "good case" was a viable, young, very ill patient whom I could diagnose and treat in a heroic manner. Rose was not that patient. She was old, confused, and easy to treat.

Not long after she was stabilized, her daughter arrived. Amid the typical ICU background of blinking lights and the rhythmic sound of ventilator bellows, we chatted about the circumstances that led up to this event. Rose was seventy-nine years old. In the jargon of the day, Rose was "just an old raisin," dry and wrinkled. Yet in spite of her advanced age, she had been extremely disruptive at the nursing home, uncooperative at bedtime, insisting that the lights be left on so she could rummage through reams of papers late into the night. In her well-worn dress, she wandered the halls of the home at all hours without regard to where she was walking, her disheveled, thin gray hair flying about. She was always preoccupied. Constant lip smacking and mumbling disturbed her roommates. Her gnarled hands trembled as she shuffled through well-worn documents while her eyes shone like black marbles—the appearance of a mad old crow.

This behavior began to annoy the nursing staff as well as some of the less demented patients. Finally, the nighttime nursing staff decided to contact the nursing home physician, who, in turn, prescribed increasing amounts of tranquilizers to quiet Rose down. Sedation depressed her breathing and lowered her blood pressure, which decreased oxygen flow to her tissues. Paradoxically, this made her more agitated, and calls were made for increased sedation, with the result leading to air hunger. This explained her heart attack. With the story sorted out to my satisfaction and with the patient stabilized by means of fluid resuscitation and medications, I felt my job was done. But to pass time, I asked Rose's daughter about the papers that were the subject of Rose's obsessive interest. She told me they were articles her mother had written plus a multitude of letters received by her over the years.

Rose was a survivor of the Armenian genocide, during which hundreds of thousands of Armenians were massacred by the Turks around the time of World War I, prior to the liberalizing reforms promoted by Ataturk. I knew little of this event for which the term *genocide* was coined. I wasn't sure if I had slept through that part of my world history class or if it had been glossed over by teachers almost as ignorant as I was. If it had been taught to me, then the basic facts had no doubt been dryly recited in a dull lecture. All that I was able to recall about that time and place was the glorious history of the Ottoman Empire and the exploits of Lawrence of Arabia. But as her daughter shared some of the details with me, I realized Rose had a story that would shock and captivate any high school class.

While sitting next to the bedside, I had the opportunity to listen to Rose's story as her daughter described the horrors experienced by victims of the jihad to rid Turkey of Christians. It dramatically took me into a world I never knew existed. And while drinking coffee, periodically looking at Rose's heart rhythm on the cardiac monitor, listening to the story, I felt transported in the same way as I had been during my first delivery and first surgery.

Rose, a child of fourteen at that time, suffered enormously. Sixty-nine members of her family were murdered. A pregnant cousin was sliced in two, and her parents were buried alive. As a young teenager, Rose was a witness yet was saved by a priest of the Armenian Apostolic Church in Marash, Turkey, who gave her sanctuary. Claiming to be sixteen and old enough for nursing school, Rose was accepted to a German Hilfsbund Mission and trained as a nurse at the German Hospital of Marash (Germany and Turkey were allies during World War I). After Germany lost the war, she joined the Armenian Medical Delegation of Marash in Adana, Turkey, where she continued working as a surgical nurse with the International Red Cross. (The British and French were occupying the area after the end of the war.) She put in long, hard hours. One night around midnight, while working, Rose and another nurse were approached by a knife-wielding French soldier who attempted to rape them. He didn't. They killed him with his own knife pulled across his throat. They vowed to maintain their silence as to which of them did it. Rose kept the secret even after her friend died at an old age. Her daughter showed me a photo of Rose as a nurse. She was stunning, with beautiful dark eyes and long black hair, seemingly no relation to the wrinkled, demented cardiac patient lying hooked to life support. As my daughter commented when she heard her story and saw her picture, "This raisin was once a luscious grape."

In spite of, or because of, her experiences, Rose had been inspired to write. She wrote many articles, published in the Armenian press, as reminders of the genocide. She sent off letters to world leaders proposing world peace and received signed responses from David Ben-Gurion,

Gamal Abdel Nasser, Charles de Gaulle, Golda Meir, and Presidents Roosevelt, Truman, Eisenhower, Johnson, and Nixon (Kennedy didn't live long enough to respond, or didn't choose to). There were even letters from Stalin and Hitler. They were all cordial letters promising to heed her advice. These were her papers. She could have been engulfed in bitterness, she could have ranted for years, she could have become suicidal—instead she wrote and, lately, shuffled papers. As her daughter finished this astonishing story, a nurse rushed up to inform me of an urgent situation with another patient—a patient who was young and extremely ill for whom I felt I might be involved in the heroic manner I thought was my calling.

As I rushed off to the trauma patient down the hall, I signed out to the next group of doctors: "There's an old demented cardiac patient in bed 3. She's just about ready for transfer."

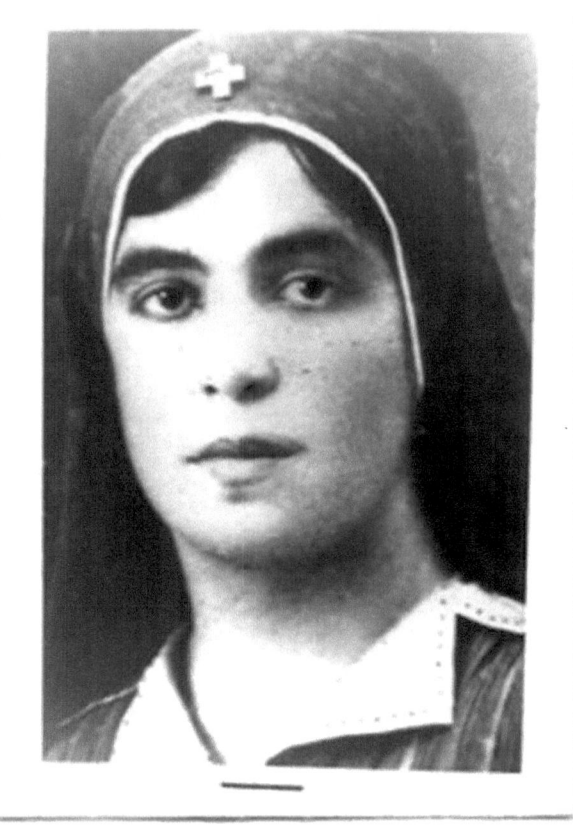

MRS. ROSE APRIGIAN
(nee MIRIAM KURDOGHLI)

Only in retrospect do I have an understanding of what a patient like Rose brings to each personal encounter. It was after that curt dismissal that I was moved to ultimately reflect upon and appreciate my patients as they serve to show us where we all fit in the world. It was this opportunity that led to my decision to dig deeper, listen more carefully, and learn from my patients. I was becoming aware of the blurred line between callousness and professional distance. Collecting stories helped to bridge the gulf between clinical judgment and empathic care.

I once heard a physician comment, "When our better instincts are suppressed, isn't that the beginning of brutality?" "Brutality" might be going a little far, but from my experience listening to the stories of my patients, I've discovered how much compassion and empathy have been lost in our complex and impersonal modern health-care system. As the process unfolded, a certain degree of continuity developed, and stories were revealed to me. I was being taught by my patients.

And thus started a succession of office visits, which prompted me to record interviews, take photos, and obtain patient releases as the taped conversations were transcribed by my children, who are proficient typists. I became privy to a remarkable collection of stories, which would have been lost had I not regretted the oversight of dehumanizing a patient by not passing on the very personal information from a patient story, Rose's story, which would have served to teach colleagues and provide for better, more humane care.

Initially, as a young doctor, the excitement of medicine and the explosion of new information were enough to keep me busy and stimulated. It helped me make it past those moments when I feared brain worms and such things, and it was all I needed as I trained in the science of medicine. I was thrilled with the reliable knowledge of science, which I felt trumped almost all other aspects of life. I had entered the profession with the focused enthusiasm typical of medical students and couldn't picture an alternative way of life. Medicine seemed to be all that was necessary to create a workable civilization, so I kept at it, building for the "greater tomorrow" that science and technology promise. It is now, armed with years of experience, that I realize that youth is, in fact, not wasted on the young; the inexperience is a virtue, and with each new experience comes a succession of revelations that produce growth.

Like learning the alphabet before learning to read, medical students must learn basic science before seeing their first patient. Once students have mastered basic science, they are exposed to medical cases and are encouraged to think of patients as little more than a collection of symptoms. The person with the disease is almost inconsequential; it has to be that way in order to function as a newly minted doctor. But then, as medical knowledge becomes hardwired, the whole person, like a larval emergence, appears from the case. As medical students, we are enthusiastic pupils, enthralled by each new case, then we are hit with little awakening shocks along the way—each patient's story serving as a jolt—and we are led further, until the larva becomes either the botfly or the butterfly, and it pops out, exposing us to something surprising and illuminating. It takes that awakening to develop a more comprehensive understanding of both our patients and ourselves.

Medical students, meeting a patient for the first time, are taught to take a careful history with the intent of obtaining information about the illness ("what's wrong?") as well as the history of past medical problems. These interviews are supposed to be recorded in the exact words of the patient in order to avoid confusion or reporter bias. Often, knowing the history described by the patient gives a clue as to the diagnosis of the disease. For example, when a patient complains of chest pain, you ask when it occurs, what precipitates it, and what relieves it. This can get more detailed with particular associated symptoms as well as lists of other related medical problems and is complemented by picking up information gleaned from family history. Taking a history opens a window into the patient's problem. For a new medical student, this is a painstaking process and can take hours to accomplish. Even then, an inexperienced student can miss important parts of the history. Lacking the intuitive intelligence developed by years of practice, they collect both the wheat and the chaff, unable to separate useful information from irrelevant details. It's not unusual to see the student, not knowing what is pertinent, refer to pages of questions geared toward particular disease entities. But after years of practice, the gathering of important details can be accomplished in a matter of minutes during the course of a seemingly innocuous conversation. You really know what to home in on after you've done this thousands of times, yet at first, as a student, you only get tidbits of information and hope for the best. Sometimes just getting a small amount of information, a little snippet of history, will allow your imagination to run wild, and you can follow it in any number of wrong directions. Eventually, you can get on track.

I was gratified to note that a change occurred and patients began to appear mixing history plus personal information with their disease processes. Before I knew it, they were giving me history lessons.

CHANCE FIRST MEETING

I first met Rudolph in the summer of 1981 when he came in for advice about a bizarre set of problems: a rash, joint swelling, and chest pain. I was thirty-two, and this fifty-five-year-old man seemed ancient to me. He had a regal demeanor and, in spite of the rash, was quite comfortable in his own skin. I determined that the chest pain that bothered him was a heart attack, and the rash and joint swelling were due to a reaction to a homeopathic medication remedy, which Rudolph had taken in an attempt to treat his chest pain. The medication caused an abnormal production of protective proteins, which would usually be formed in order to fight attacks from foreign substances. Our bodies have this defense mechanism to protect us from foreign invaders like bacteria. When harmful bacteria enter the body, it triggers an attack by millions of small protector proteins, and the bacteria are destroyed. The reason our own cells aren't attacked is that "sentry" proteins stand guard and ward off such destruction. Some of these weapons made by our bodies' own defensive network are called antibodies. In this case, they misfired, and the sentry was overpowered. The antibodies fought against Rudolph's cells and body tissues, creating a rash and acute arthritis. I was able to effectively treat this and felt the office visit with Rudolph would be short and sweet.

Seated in my office, I peered at him over a pile of medical charts while the radio played unobtrusive classical music as background for what I expected to be a routine patient interview. As we spoke—and as I tried to figure things out—I became distracted by his thick German accent and redirected my questions to his life history. He told me he had come from Germany to America in 1946 and had taken a job on a farm in Kansas. The tenor of the conversation was changing, and I, a Jew, tensed imperceptibly. I assumed the worst: he must be an escaped Nazi, and I would be expected to treat him. As in the novel *Horcynus Orca*, in which a soldier accidentally winds up needing the help of his victims, I considered how privileged I was to find myself there, in a situation so rich, rare, and fortunate, and how privileged I was to have what I believed to be a Nazi needing my help. I knew that Hippocrates had developed the doctor's code: to treat all patients without prejudice. Yet the idea of treating a Nazi was among one of the most complicated issues that I could imagine. Their terrifying behavior set the standard for modern barbarism, and I did not feel that I owed them any medical care. I wondered whether I could overlook what was implied by the Hippocratic Oath; I wasn't sure how I could handle treating a Nazi. Hippocrates was an ancient Greek; what did he know from Nazis?

I couldn't get it out of my mind and decided to probe deeper, expecting to react the moment he admitted his dark background; then I would expose him for what he was. Indeed, his background was dark, but not at all what I had anticipated.

His mother was American and from a wealthy and devout Christian family. His father's side came from Spain around the time of the Inquisition. The family name was Nathan—they were Jewish. At that time, Jews either converted to Catholicism, were exiled, or were killed. The Nathans chose exile and left Spain for Hamburg during the height of the Inquisition. They changed their name from Nathan to H. and started a banking business in Germany and England. Jews were limited by law to very few occupations, and banking was one of them. I no longer felt compelled to expose him as a monster. I sat back and listened.

Rudolph's grandfather, with a letter of introduction from a British bank, moved to Berlin in 1881 (one hundred years before this encounter) and opened a bank. He married and became very involved with the German culture—Goethe, Schiller, and Wagner—and a part of an integrated German society. He was related to the Mendelssohn family. Lessing, a famous German poet, wrote a play called *Nathan der Weise* (*Nathan the Wise*) about Rudolph's great-uncle Moses Mendelssohn. To this day, there is a Mendelssohn society in Berlin, which tries to encourage enlightened thought.

Rudolph's father became a colonial administrator in German African colonies, now Tanzania. But after World War I, Germany lost its colonies. He sold some banks, traveled to Africa to hunt big game, and bought large tracts of German farmland, which is why Rudolph grew up on a large farming estate.

The family felt discriminated against during the 1930s, yet they were unsure how much the sentiment would increase. The Nazis were powerful, and Rudolph found it disorienting to see the growth of such a hate-filled, irrational doctrine. He told me he felt distant from it: "It was as though it were happening to somebody else." Not all Germans were impressed with Hitler. In fact, in 1932, the German president, Field Marshal Hindenburg, reacted to meeting Hitler with the comment "That man for Chancellor? I'll make him a postmaster and he can lick stamps with my head on them." However, Hindenburg soon recanted; like others, he fell in line.

As a child, Rudolph saw the storm troopers come (the SA wore brown shirts while the elite guards wore black shirts and were called SS) and, initially, found them silly in their funny brown uniforms and swastikas. Once, he stood in a crowd, listening to Hitler speak. He thought the Fuhrer charismatic and noted that people responded to him enthusiastically. "There's a feeling when you're in a mass of people that's hard to resist, and you want to shout," he said. "It's very difficult not to, but I tried not to. If you ask me whether I could feel the sense of wanting to join in, I would say yes."

In 1933, Rudolph went to school in Berlin, but that didn't work out because discrimination against the Jews had started. He couldn't participate in most activities because he was considered Jewish. He was banned from joining in athletics with "pure Germans." Government functionaries informed him that he was a Mischling—half Jewish. It was the first time he learned his father's family was Jewish. The family began to suffer a series of insults. There were servants in their enormous home, but the female servants were not permitted to live in the house because Rudolph's father was Jewish. So Rudolph, at age twelve, to avoid both prejudice and embarrassment, was taken out of the school and sent to England, where the family still had relatives. His aunt Alice decided he should go to a Benedictine Catholic school because the food was better. Aunt Alice was a big woman who liked good food very much (her brothers had gone to Eton, and the food there was terrible). In spite of all this, Rudolph still felt a strong fondness for Germany, and during the 1936 Olympics, he felt proud of the German heavyweight boxer Max Schmeling. Like many Germans, he felt Schmeling represented something strong and successful about him as a German citizen, in spite of the fact that German Jews were ostracized within their own country.

In the meantime, his father, back in Germany, lost his hunting license because he was a Jew. It was one of a series of debasements, and he did not grasp what was happening to him, his family, and his community. Devastated and humiliated by the experience—he had felt quite assimilated into German society and couldn't comprehend the dramatic change in his status—he suffered a fatal heart attack.

Rudolph was summoned home to Germany; he was now the male head of household, a perverse sort of bar mitzvah for the thirteen-year-old Rudolph.

It was around this dark time that he learned to appreciate jazz: "A few of us used to sneak around and listen to jazz because it was American and represented freedom. This was dangerous but, in a way, quite liberating. My cousin was a pianist and would play a jazzed-up version of the Horst Wessel song."

I didn't know what Rudolph was talking about and mentioned that I had never heard of that song. "Was it the horse whistle song?"

"No," he continued, "the Horst Wessel song was the Nazi national anthem. When my cousin played the jazzed-up version at different venues, it would make us laugh because this seemed like such a clever form of rebellion. Whenever it was played, we smiled and shared knowing glances with each other. The Nazis executed my cousin for this."

I looked across my desk at the top of Rudolph's bowed head.

During this period, Rudolph's mother's family entreated them to come to America, but by 1939, Jewish families had difficulty emigrating. Rudolph had to sign up for the military. He was then identified as a Jew and forced to register as a Mischling. This meant that he would soon be transported to a labor camp. The SS (the "black shirts") went to his family home and said, "You can't stay here." They confiscated the home because of the Jewish bloodlines.

At this moment, the radio announcer's voice returned, startling me, and I realized I'd been so engrossed in Rudolph's story that I'd lost track of the music, the files piled on my desk, and the ordinary sounds of daily life outside my office door. And quite unexpectedly, I was realizing another aspect to the practice of medicine: the person within the patient and how it affects the way I practice medicine.

"Then I went to work at a stove-making factory," Rudolph continued. He was looking at his hands folded in his lap, and it occurred to me that his eyes hadn't met mine since he'd begun his story. "There was a formal setup with the Labor Office. However, the registration office was bombed, and Jews were told to reregister with the police. My uncle advised me not to reregister, so I didn't."

His uncle, oddly enough, did reregister ("Maybe to protect me," Rudolph said, but he never really knew why) and subsequently perished in a concentration camp. Rudolph, by virtue of not having reregistered, had erased any trace of where and who he really was. His mother and sister moved to one of their family homes in the mountains "with the help of Aryan friends." Rudolph, after quite some time, made his way to the mountain home and was reunited with his mother and sister. By then, the Russians were rolling through eastern Germany. The Russian army took over the eastern German lands and property from the SS. This included all the estate and farmland that were owned by Rudolph's family.

Finally, the Americans arrived. Because Rudolph's mother was American and registered with the Red Cross, the American soldiers were looking for her cottage in the hope of finding an American war survivor. When the soldiers arrived at her cottage, General Gay stepped out of the jeep and introduced himself, explained that American troops now occupied Himmler's house (Himmler, the SS commander, was considered one of Hitler's architects of the war and of the annihilation of the Jews), and now invited Rudolph's family to a party thrown by General Patton, who was leading the American efforts in Germany. Rudolph was offered and accepted a job working for General Patton in Himmler's house. Yet he knew he would have to leave Germany. The Russians occupied Rudolph's family's property in what was to become East Germany. Because Rudolph no longer could return to the family home, he was placed in a refugee camp along with those who had been liberated from concentration camps. It was the first meeting he had with those with tattoos (the tattoos placed as numbers to identify the Jews) and his first contact with Jewish culture. Rudolph recalled, "There was an intense sense of community and sharing. It took a long time for them to realize that there was no longer rationing. They were bound together by tattoos, by a degree of alienation from society, and by betrayal by their countries." However, the Jewish refugees eventually found a renewed sense of hope, which, for many, mingled with the despair that they somehow overcame, permitted them to survive.

With difficulty typical of the times, Rudolph arranged transport to the United States where he worked on the family farm in Kansas before furthering his education in Boston. He still sits on the board of directors of banks in Berlin. For over forty years, he had tried unsuccessfully to regain ownership of the family property in Germany. Then the Berlin Wall fell, and lands that had been confiscated by the SS were returned to their owners. Rudolph became one of the largest landholders in all of Germany. He said, "When I got the land back, my kids asked why I didn't jump up and down. I don't know. I'm not that type. I'm more reserved. Maybe it's something else. You never get everything back."

The heart attack, rash, and arthritis were treated and are a distant memory, but the story remains with Rudolph and, now, with me. Treating his disease was the easy part—it was gratifying. Facing issues of personal integrity made a bigger impact and, in many ways, led to greater understanding of the human condition. Like his Mendelssohn ancestors, Rudolph continues to encourage enlightened thought, impart wisdom, and carry on the tradition of educating those who listen.

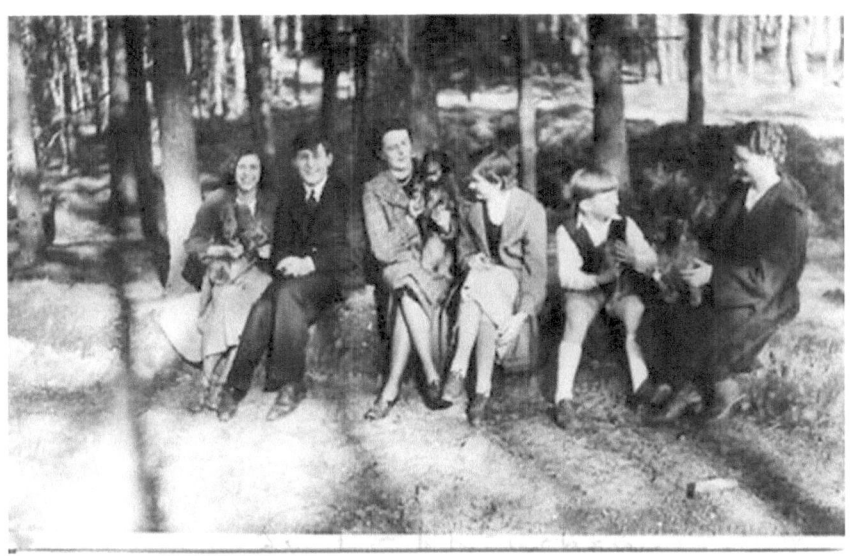

Rudolph, second from the left, with family members

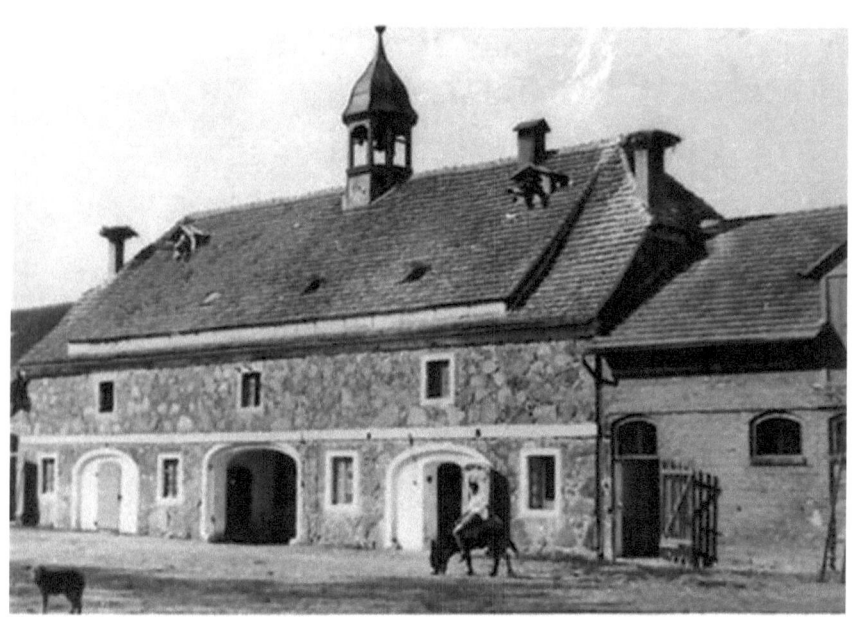

The stables at the country estate

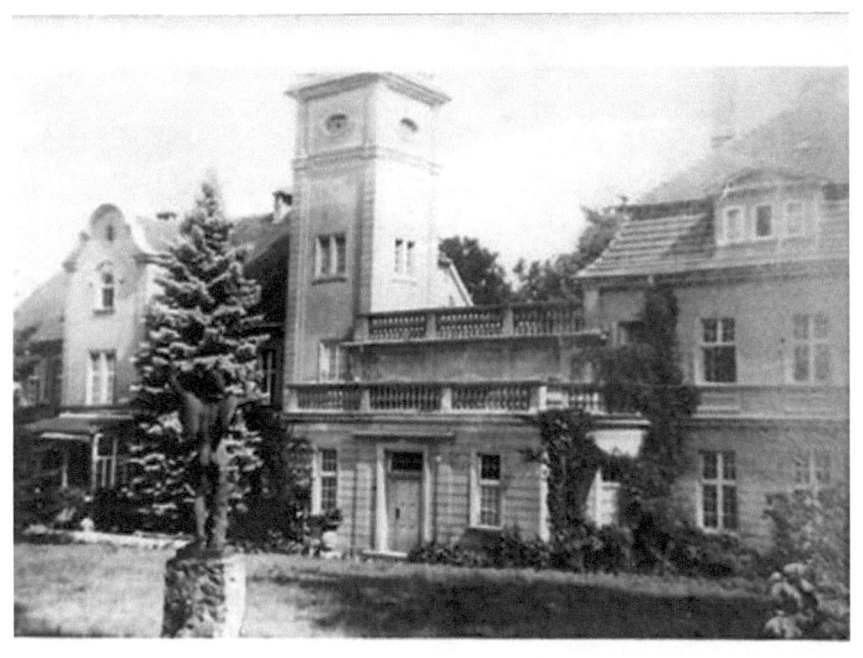

Rudolph's family's country home in Germany

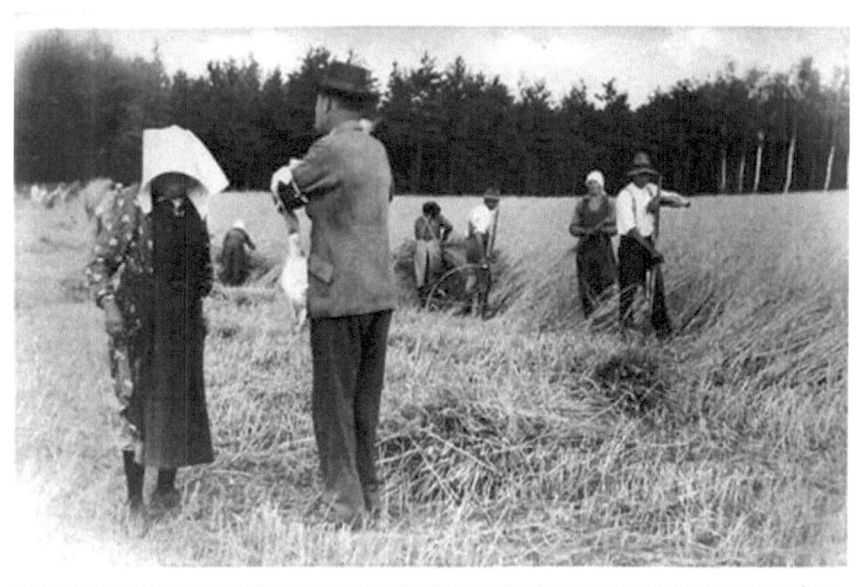

Workers at harvest on Rudolph's family estate

Physicians are in a unique position: we gather medical information, and we witness the breakdown and repair of the body. But if we take time, along the way, to gather stories and histories as well, we can also witness the breakdown and repair of the human spirit. Often the stories have not been told before, but are told in safety, in part, because of the protective nature of the situation, alone with the doctor they trust. And there exists the strong desire to get it out. Like the excision of a tumor or an infected foreign body, it will be removed, leaving a not-quite-empty space. The stories told to the doctor provide historical information, and a physician, distancing himself from the event, may gain perspective. This perspective can help the patient or may simply educate the listener. It takes time to digest and process the story, yet it is very important for there to be a listener, hopefully one who will not abandon them once the story is told. It is then that a remarkable transformation occurs and the young doctor becomes aware of the human within the case. The result is a more complete sense of the patient and a better understanding of the world they come from, the world we all share.

As the listener, I found my knowledge evolved as a unique view of human nature and the human predicament developed. I have been struck by human resiliency and ability to cope in the face of adversity. For me, this also creates a new dynamic where the bond with the patient tightens.

THE STAMP COLLECTOR'S FAMILY

"It was an eerie sensation, at night, pitch-black in the middle of the ocean: silence interrupted only by the *glub, glub, glub* sound of German and British U-boats rising up through the still, dark, uncertain ocean surface," Anna M. recounted. The banana boat had left from its port in Lisbon in December 1939, its cargo, the escaping Jews on their way to America. The boat captain had never sailed the boat past the Azores but had agreed on a price to take them to their destination. The M. family, Mr. and Mrs. M with their eleven-year-old daughter and thirteen-year-old boy, had little more than their life jackets and high hopes. The boat almost made it without damage, but a winter storm caused it to bounce like a floating package and drift for days, disrupting propellers and navigation. The M. family finally arrived in New York on January 8, 1940. I met Anna M. and her daughter fifty years later, when the pain from an inflamed facial nerve brought the older woman to my attention.

They were from Cologne, Germany, where Mr. M had been arrested on trumped-up charges in 1933 but managed to bribe his way out of jail. An insidious national change was occurring: intellectuals, physicians, and lawyers were not allowed to practice in their professions if they were Jewish. On November 9, 1938, the massive pogrom known as Kristallnacht began, and thousands of Jewish businesses were destroyed and uncountable numbers of Jews were slaughtered or incarcerated. On

November 10, Mr. M. was arrested, again, and sent to Buchenwald (one of the first concentration camps). He was fortunate, after a period of time, that his Catholic business associate was able to convince authorities that he needed Mr. M. to help turn over their factory to the Nazis. Instead, the associate smuggled Mr. M. over the border into Belgium and eventually arranged to hide Mrs. M. and the two children under a car seat and get them into Belgium. The business associate was never heard from again but was last reported to be under arrest by the Nazis.

"Some Jews were able to go to Palestine, but the sad fact was that the world did not want the refugees. There was nowhere to go, and the Depression was affecting everyone," Mrs. M. told me. "It was a way of life, which no one could believe, as if someone today would come up to you and tell you that this would happen to a segment of your society. You would tell them to go away, it is inconceivable, and somebody is going to come to their senses."

Adolf Hitler promised to build up the country and put everyone to work. The Nazis took everything away from the Jews and became rich overnight, and that helped flame the fires of greed and hatred.

On May 10, the Germans invaded Belgium, and the M. family joined throngs of people trying to cross the Maginot Line (on the border between France and Germany) because they believed the Germans would not invade France. What initially seemed unimaginable became routine; packing whatever could be carried, the refugees began walking in a crowd that moved like migrating animals. They were starving and walked amid bombing, planes diving and strafing, and all the horrors of war, often ignoring bodies along the side of the road and seeing women carrying dead babies, the desperate search for a family member, and the weeping. The staggering crowd began to look peculiarly alike, until the planes would begin their indiscriminate attacks, and amid the panic, direct hits were identified by bloody corpses. At the French border, they were identified as Germans and could not explain that, as Jews, they were "not part of this." They were placed in a camp with German prisoners of war. "It was preposterous," Mrs. M. said.

The German troops arrived and liberated the prisoners of war, permitting the M. family to escape again. They hid in various homes and farms, finally making it to Portugal. They were lucky. "A large part of the family was lost in Auschwitz," Anna M. whispered as she looked out the window at nothing. She said she was grateful to have her daughter still with her. "You must have a daughter," she added.

Mr. M. is a philatelist and had put together a postal history of the Holocaust in response to the questions his teenage children asked him about family members lost in concentration camps. Yet he never spoke of his own experience in Buchenwald. Like his Jewish ancestors, he struggled with self-conquest and never with self-analysis. Mrs. M. said that her husband dealt with the burden of loss by doing research, whereas she felt that it was a blessing to survive and that she did not want to pass on hate or to fall apart. She told me, "There are moments when the memories trickle and creep in. I trust that this inflamed nerve is not about to open a crack and allow for a flood."

I couldn't answer. I'm sure it's a coincidence that my daughter, born shortly after this interview, is named Anna.

Victims of Nazi Germany
Postal History

Konzentrationslager Dachau K 3

Meine Anschrift:
Name: Skibinski Wladislaus
Geboren am: 11 März 1903
Gef.-Nr. 11056 Block 12/2

Dachau, den 30.III.41.

Liebe Eltern u. Schwester!

Euren Brief vom 24.III.41. habe ich am 28.III.41. erhalten. Er hat mir viel Freude gemacht, weil ich von Euch schon lange keinen Brief erhalten habe. Es freut mich auch sehr liebe Eltern, dass alles bei euch liebe Eltern ist, dass Vater arbeitet und alls schön

Instructions include: "visits to camp are forbidden.....inquiries are useless.....packages may not be sent, as everything can be bought here.....". Faded camp censor cachet, same as used on outside cover, also appears on inside page of letter sheet (not visible).

Victims of Nazi Germany
Postal History

EXODUS TO CUBA

As economic and social conditions became more and more unbearable for German Jews in 1939, urgent attempts were made to emigrate by whatever means possible. Strict national quota systems abroad made the leaving of Germany most difficult and frustrating.

On 13 May 1939, 930 German Jews who had bought passage and secured landing certificates from the Cuban Government, sailed from HAMBURG on the German ship "St. Louis", destination HAVANA, CUBA. Most of these refugees had been promised eventual entry into the USA on the basis of fulfilling U.S. immigration requirements in Germany.

On 27 May 1939 the "St. Louis" docked at HAVANA, but only to find that Cuba would not permit the passengers entry. The ransom price for a sanctuary in Cuba was $500,000 in cash. Frantic negotiations finally broke down after neighboring countries, including the USA, failed to help. The ship's German captain had no choice, and so he reluctantly ordered the "St. Louis" return trip to Hamburg.

The governments of Belgium, Holland, France and England offered a haven for the passengers at the last moment and the "St. Louis" discharged its human cargo at ANTWERP, Belgium on 17 June 1939.

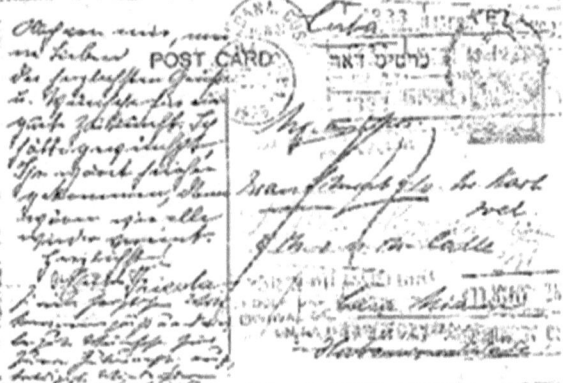

The above background helps in introducing this card sent from TEL AVIV, Palestine on 5 June 1939 as a "welcome greeting" to a Jewish couple scheduled to arrive in HAVANA on a second such planned voyage on board the German ship "Orinoco". However as a result of the fiasco of the "St. Louis", this ship was recalled to Hamburg after only several days on the high seas. All its passengers were made to return to their points of origin. The addressees of this card, and his wife, may never to have subsequently perished in AUSCHWITZ.

Letter to a Jewish couple escaping from Europe, expecting to arrive in Cuba on the ship the *Saint Louis*, but sent back to certain death

As I learned more and more about my patients, the insurance network was demanding that I do less and less because that would result in increased profits for the insurer. They claimed to be reducing waste. They had hired numerous nurses, doctors, and other administrators at great costs to search high and low for sources of waste, but it struck me that one man's waste was another man's dinner. The insurance executives were certainly not starving. The insurance requirement was to reduce testing as well as reject prescriptions for costly drugs and referrals. They also insisted that medical records be put on a computer ostensibly to share information with other doctors (a fine concept), but particularly to share information with the insurer (a disturbing reality). The overwhelming reliance on computers resulted in the attitude to do less and listen less, because it was just data on a computer screen, not a person needing the best of the doctor's skill and compassion.

LOSING WORDS

Eric M. was frail when I first met him almost twenty years before his death. He had had four major heart attacks and many minor ones (handling each cardiac crisis with quiet dignity in an attempt to prevent worry among his loved ones). After the death of his first wife, he remarried a woman who would invariably describe him as a kind, soft-spoken gentleman. I agreed with that assessment. Eric's only concern was a fear of losing his words. He chose his words carefully and always expected to have a multitude to choose from.

He was Jewish, born in Vienna and, when he was old enough, worked for his father, who was an architect and a builder. After his father's death, Eric and his three younger brothers took over the business until a few days after Hitler "liberated" Austria. Their longtime business manager happened to be a covert Nazi, and the new government permitted him to take over the business. Four uniformed SA brown shirts with swastika armbands entered the office, pointed pistols at Eric's chest, and ordered him to open the safe. They took all of the safe's contents and then drove away in Eric's car. As Eric spoke with a soft, measured speech, he recalled an unforgettable scene where two Catholic female employees fell on their knees, crying and clasping their hands in prayer, pleading, "Don't kill him, don't kill him." The Nazis let him live, but after this traumatic episode, his days were saturated with fear.

A car stopping in front of the house or the sudden unexpected ringing of the doorbell was a frightening experience.

Then, in the early morning of May 28, 1938, two plainclothes policemen arrived at the building where his office had been located and where he had a small apartment. He was taken to the police station and, from there, to the train with many other Jewish men. While running to the train, they were beaten mercilessly by SS soldiers shouting humiliations. The night trip on the train was a grotesque nightmare, but the destination was a greater nightmare: Dachau. Over the entrance gate of the concentration camp was the inscription "Arbeit macht frei" ("Work will make you free"). This reminded Eric of the first words in the Haggadah (the story of Exodus told at Passover), "The Egyptians oppressed the Israelites with harsh labor and made their lives bitter."

Eric's hair was shorn; he was given a prison uniform and forced to stand for hours before he was sent to the barracks. He fainted, but a political prisoner, whose name he never learned, carried him on his shoulders to the barracks and waited with him until he sufficiently aroused (thereby saving his life). At the barracks, he saw toilets with bread piled in them, and Eric started to cry as prisoners hungrily dug in. His "lifesaver" consoled him by saying, "You too will get used to it." He never thought that he would eat the bread soaked in the urinal, but he did. At Dachau, he worked sixteen hours a day and, in my office, broke down weeping when he described how he survived. He noted that he got out before the gas chambers and ovens were in full use. He was released, thanks to a devoted cousin who went to Buchenwald, with letters and money, to arrange for a visa so Eric could go to America (which had not yet entered the war). By then, much of his family had dispersed or was lost. His four sisters and his mother were killed in Auschwitz.

He arrived in the United States by boat and recalled the intense emotional experience of passing the Statue of Liberty, which is inscribed with the words "I lift my lamp beside the golden door." He entered the country that gave him his freedom and permitted him to live the dreams he dared to dream. Thus, he tries to not to forget the words he first spoke on American soil: "God bless America."

He believed his heart was strong because it had survived much worse than simple lack of coronary blood flow. It had survived a heaviness of heart brought on by loss and as a witness that was greater than disease itself. That knowledge had enabled him to get through his heart attacks with such aplomb. But he was worried—he did not want to lose the words to tell his story.

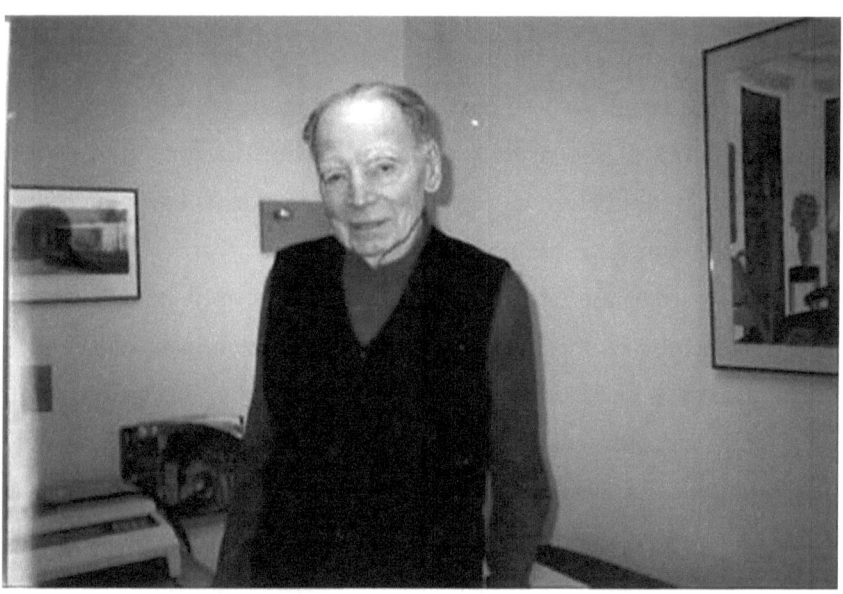

Konzentrationslager Buchenwald
Kommandantur

Weimar-Buchenwald, den 27. Jan. 1939

Entlassungsschein

Der Schutzhäftling ... Erich M...rek
geb. ... ... hat vom 3.6.38

... ...

... ... 26.1.39

... ... entlassen.

Der Lagerkommandant

SS-Hauptsturmführer

Translation

Copy

Concentration Camp Buchenwald   Weimar-Buchenwald
Office of the Commander   January 27, 1939

Letter of Release

The protective prisoner ...EW ERICH M...REK, born May 17, 1907 in Vienna, was returned to concentration camp ... ... in custody from June 3, 1938 to this day by order of the Gestapo on January 26, 1939, and was returned to Vienna.

The Commander of the Camp

s/ SS Chief Storm Leader

TATTOO

Mack A.'s diffuse arthritis caused him pain and stiffness in multiple joints, and his diabetes brought on nerve damage, numbness, and tingling in his feet. When he hobbled into my office, his small faded-blue eyes hiding beneath puffy lids were filled with sadness, and he spoke with the thick Polish accent he had been unable to shake even after forty years in Boston. His pain increased over the weekend, and he was concerned that his medical problems were worsening.

Pain triggers are often clear—injury, nerve damage, diminished blood flow, tumor, toxins, or joint swelling—but sometimes the cause is more subtle. My gaze drifted from his face to the number tattooed on his left arm as he started to tell his story. He witnessed the era in our history when the Nazis consumed the Jews, starting with the children and infirm, then the rest.

Mack had the misfortune to have been born in Plonsk, Poland, about sixty kilometers from Warsaw. On September 30, 1939, the Germans attacked Poland and, two weeks later, entered Plonsk. With no resistance from the city, the Germans ordered all Jews into a corner of the city and called it a ghetto, and no one stopped them. Those rounded up were bewildered since they believed that they were still accepted as members of society in spite of growing disaffection among the Christians toward the Jews. The Jews were forced to wear a yellow star over their left breast and a yellow star on the back; those who were rebellious or ignorant enough to appear without their yellow star were shot. Some people were caught outside the ghetto trying to find food or shoes, and they too were shot.

A few weeks later, the Germans ordered all Jews to fill out papers cataloguing what they owned. Rifles were placed to the heads of Jews, and they were told to cooperate or the family would be killed; sometimes a shot would be fired, and a body would crumple. The A. family had a tailor shop and had to inventory their machines, their scissors, their thread, everything. What seemed to be an innocuous request was actually an ominous, threatening gesture proving to all that the Nazis were in charge. This process was repeated throughout the ghetto. Then the Germans arrested one hundred Jews and put them in jail; these hostages could be exchanged for a million zlotys or be shot. Relatives asked everybody they knew for money to save their family members. Mack and his family felt the communal sense of panic and contributed what they could. The Germans got the money, but the people were shot anyway.

Today there is a grave outside of Auschwitz bearing their names. As he spoke, Mack leaned forward slightly, staring at the piles of charts on my desk. Strains from a piece by Mahler, or maybe it was Wagner, played on the office radio. My gaze drifted back to Mack's face.

Mack was seventeen when thousands of SS men with machine guns and German shepherds surrounded the ghetto and began taking Jews from the city. They knocked open doors and windows, yelling, "Rads, Juden" ("Come out, Jews") and chased people onto the street, hitting and beating and shooting. "People were pushed, beaten, stabbed, or shot." Then the trucks came, loaded up the Jews, and took them to a concentration camp called Stavica (where the prisoners made ammunition and springs for trains). Mack worked in a small room with high-pressure machines, pressing hot iron to form springs. Occasionally, the machines could develop an air pocket and explode, shooting pieces of metal like bullets. Once, while Mack was working with a fellow prisoner who was a bit slow, the SS man operating the press let it down on the prisoner. The prisoner almost got out, but the press caught his head, "smashing it to nothing." Mack continued to work while his tears clouded his eyes, and the SS guards laughed with cigarettes forming puffs of smoke around their smiles. Not long after that, his group was put on trains. They were bewildered and nervous since they didn't know where they were going. But they followed the commands and threats of shouting Nazi soldiers. Mack added, almost as an afterthought, "Those who did not get on trains were sent to the gas chambers, which were located nearby."

Mack traveled in a cattle car—no windows—with an oily, smelly black disinfectant on the floor. No food, no water, and after three days, half the people were dead, parents unable to save children, children unable to save parents. When the doors finally opened, he was at Auschwitz. Dozens of train tracks led to the camp, transporting thousands for daily extermination. (This was an enormous technological feat, well organized, well disciplined, and monstrous.) Hair was cut, toys were taken and placed in a pile, and shoes and valuables were removed. There were SS men and dogs all around, and on the left, seated at a table, was Dr. Mengele. He pointed to the left or right, separating those who could work from those who couldn't. Those on the left stood still while those on the right were told they were going to the showers. But it wasn't the showers; it was the gas chamber. Mack didn't know about the gas chambers at first, but he had a suspicion that something about the showers was wrong despite the sign overhead that said something about cleanliness; it should have read more like the entrance to Dante's inferno: "Abandon all hope."

People did as they were told, Mack explained, because even though it didn't feel right, they couldn't believe one human being would kill another for nothing, that an entire society would condone this, that anyone would want to kill a child, based on nothing more than a physician's finger pointing to the left or right. It was simply Dr. Mengele's finger pointing in a particular direction. All the children were gone by day 2—all of them went to the right.

The SS were helped by the Zunder commander (all those were Jews, and all were gone in six months, killed to prevent them from developing too much power). A Kapo was a Jew who worked under the Zunder commander, and Mack's cousin was a Kapo who witnessed the naked bodies after the gas crystals had hit those in the "showers." They were scratched and bloody; climbing to breathe, they had formed human pyramids, locked together in death.

The area needed to be cleaned because victims urinated and defecated as they died. The bodies needed to be examined for hidden wealth, including gold in the teeth and jewels that had been hidden in the anus. They were then removed and sent to the crematorium to make room for others. Due to the destructive nature of the toxins, bodies occasionally fell apart. The crematorium couldn't handle the load of gassed bodies and had a backlog. Mack spoke in almost a whisper as he explained that he was commanded to dig trenches for burial, including one for his brother's disfigured corpse. His cousin was given the job of looking for hidden jewels. Mack's sad blue eyes betrayed the flat, unemotional sound of his voice as he conveyed to me the story of the discovery of the death of his younger brother whom he had found among the gassed bodies. But for Mack and others, life in the camp continued.

The block boss was given the duty of feeding people and keeping the block clean, making sure no one hid and checking that everyone reported for work at Birkenau, the work camp affiliated with Auschwitz. He was top man because he controlled the food. There was black bread, thick and wet. There was soup made of potato skins (the SS men ate the potatoes and discarded the skins). The prisoners were starving, and Mack recalled a day when four young boys from the surrounding area passed bread to a few prisoners. The Nazis caught the boys, had them kneel against a wall, and shot them in the head.

"However," Mack recalled as he tried to blink away a small tear that had formed, "you would get a thin slice of salami when there were hangings." Once, a few prisoners were caught with a radio. They were desperate for news from the outside world and listened to the BBC. They had constructed the radio from airplane scraps (the Germans used the aluminum from planes that had been shot down, and they had mountains of it at the camp). The prisoners were placed on chairs with ropes around their necks—a gallows. The chairs were kicked out, the offending prisoners were hung, and salami was distributed.

Mack and others believed that someone had to escape to "bring the word out"; there was still a free world that needed to be notified about what was occurring in Auschwitz. They hid one man in an aluminum pile, thinking he would escape after the prisoners returned to Auschwitz from Birkenau, but the SS counted the prisoners according to the numbers tattooed on their forearms (Mack referred to the number tattoo on his forearm, which was an added insult to religious Jews because it defies Mosaic law against cutting or marking oneself spelled out in Deuteronomy, but it was the SS who cut/tattooed him and who knew his number, yet not his name, and he felt that he would always wear his tattoo in order to remember and, also, as an act of defiance, since he survived intact). The SS expected six hundred prisoners, but counted 599. Mack explained, "They couldn't let anyone escape. They couldn't let anyone know." The SS men made the prisoners stand around—tired, hungry, and frightened—until they found the hidden man. It was the same thing—another hanging, another piece of salami. Mack, again, gazed down with sad eyes and mumbled, "But who will be there to say if no one survives and all is forgotten?"

Mack also remembered the trains arriving from Holland and France. These weren't cattle cars. People had arrived in regular trains and had been advised to take necessities with them. The Jews disembarked at Auschwitz, carrying suitcases filled with precious items (photos, special clothes, jewelry), believing they were going to Canada. It was explained to them that they would get their possessions back after they passed through a building with the sign "Canada" on it. "First, you must take a shower," they were told.

By 1944, the war was not going well for the Germans. The Russians were coming, and the decision was made to evacuate Auschwitz. Mack's cousin, feeling all was hopeless since the SS were starting to panic and were killing more workers, tried to escape and was machine-gunned at the fence. Those remaining were to march for the next two weeks. It was bitter cold, and they lacked warm clothing, shoes, and food as they were harnessed with ropes in order to pull trucks into Austria. Those who fell or tired out were shot. Out of three million prisoners who entered Auschwitz, only twelve thousand were now left. Fewer survived the march.

Mack made it to another camp in Austria and was imprisoned with eight thousand Russians and two thousand Jews. In 1945, the SS assembled the prisoners and told them the Americans had arrived but that the prisoners would be safe in special tunnels. One of the Russians spread the word that the tunnels were filled with dynamite. Hundreds of Russians started to yell, "Nein, nein nicht gehen," which means "No, don't go." The SS were astonished. In all the years that Mack had contact with the Nazis, no one said no to an SS man. By then, Mack felt it in his heart and in his blood, and he, too, could now shout no. His words punched the air. The prisoners returned to their barracks, and the Nazis fled, but before they fled, they put elderly Austrian townspeople in their SS uniforms in case the American soldiers entered and tried to shoot the guards. Four American soldiers arrived at the camp as the "liberators." They kept saying, "What is this? We didn't expect this." They had no orders and didn't seem to know what to do, so they left.

Like many in the camp, Mack decided that he was now free. He found a bayonet and went to a village for food. He couldn't look at me, and his voice trembled as he spoke, "I am ashamed of what I did." With an observable heaviness, he reflected upon his behavior as he described how he had violently entered homes and took what he needed. Like others, he didn't know what to do next, so he returned to the camp where he saw hundreds lying in pools of blood. They had starved for so long that once they ate, their gastrointestinal tracts couldn't tolerate food and they developed bloody diarrhea, killing many of those who had survived long enough only to be destroyed by unfair retribution brought about by freedom.

Although the SS ran away, some didn't get far. They tried to disguise themselves, but they could be recognized by a small tattoo on their shoulders, and Mack thought he found one of the guards. Together with other prisoners, they tore off the guard's clothes to locate the tattoo. Once he was clearly identified, they hanged the SS guard by his feet and kicked him in the head until he died. The conquering American soldiers went by and asked, "Who did this? We have to know who killed him. A thing like that cannot be allowed!"

But Mack and the others cried, "We got justice!"

The soldiers replied, "We have to take people who commit a crime to court."

Mack yelled back, "Did the SS take us to court? Did they find us guilty? They killed millions at Auschwitz."

The alarmed and confused Americans tried to figure out what happened and took a few people in for questioning; they could not understand that a few thousand people executing orders had built a secret system of extermination and that this system had been created by a "civilized" nation. That concept too was difficult for the American soldiers to grasp.

Mack eventually moved to Boston, and I had been treating him for many years, listening to his story, which I eventually recorded. By the time he presented with the episode of severe pain, I had heard most of the details of this seminal experience. He said the pain came on suddenly, on Saturday, while he was seated in the synagogue to attend a Bat Mitzvah. He was watching the girl read from the Torah and happened to glance down at her ankle. And there he noticed a small butterfly tattoo.

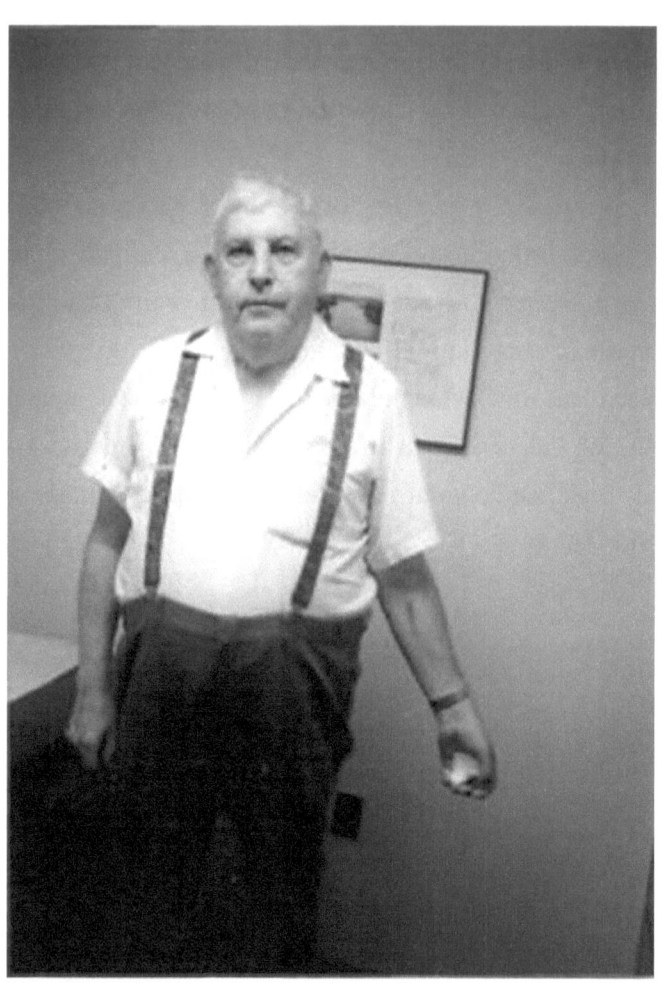

The recurrent theme of tattoos developed as I interviewed more patients. It is a particular problem for the Jew, who, from the precepts of Deuteronomy, is forbidden to scar himself. Yet scarring, in the form of internal and external tattoos, occurs. Tattoos are not only present as identifiers of Nazi death-camp survivors; they also serve as an attempt to develop a protective covering to hide the psychic ills lurking beneath the skin, in some cases placed to provide a "brave or fearsome" outer cover. In the most perverse case, they serve as a badge of honor worn by the SS who routinely committed atrocities. However, most of the marks are internal, a spiritual tattoo, which mark each person like an etching on hard metal—difficult to place but impossible to burnish off, lasting a lifetime. These internal tattoos are not limited to the patient but to the physician as well. It is the patient with their stories that always leave a mark.

The penultimate patient story, "Octopus Trap," is not simply the tale of an aging couple; it is a cautionary tale for any relationship, including doctor-patient, when familiarity leads to relaxation, where we adjust our preconceived notions and no longer rely on "blink of an eye" interaction. Thus, to relax within that relationship is part of being human, but it is also the essential trap within that necessary bond. Although the interpersonal bond makes for smoother interaction, it makes for a difficult release. From youth to age, the experience of developing a deep relationship is an enormous part of what makes us who we are.

It keeps coming back to the stories, not just what we learn from them, but also what they represent. As one patient put it, "In the end, who will I recognize and who will know me? Whose story can I remember, and who will remember mine?" He softly spoke, "I worry that the world has been closing in around the space I used to occupy. What will remain? The vapor and the story is all that is left." We can do worse than to be the keeper of the stories.

APOLOGY

I used to work a couple of summer vacation weeks each year in the emergency room on Martha's Vineyard. It was there, in the mid-1980s, that I met Petros (although he didn't ask, I have chosen not to use his real name). He was on vacation and had slipped and fallen out of a loft, resulting in a long gash in his side. I placed a dozen sutures and gave him a tetanus shot. He was beefy and bent, with sad, unreflective eyes and sparse gray hair, and he spoke broken English. He told me he was returning to Boston around the time I was and asked if he could go to my office there in order to get his stitches removed. We made the appointment.

On the designated day, he showed up early, giving us extra time together before my other scheduled appointments. Since I was recording stories from World War II veterans, I asked if he had been in Europe during the war. He said that he had and agreed to have his story recorded and signed a release but added that his tale probably wouldn't be very interesting. He said he was from Romania, and in fact, his brother had been the minister of something-or-other in Romania during the war. He told me that the Romanians weren't sure which side of the war to be on, but because the king had a Jewish mistress whom they all detested, they chose the Germans.

Petros became an army captain, thanks to his family connections. He was in charge of the troops the day the harbor in his hometown, on the Black Sea coast, was mined, a Romanian army headquarters in

Odessa was blown up, and a bunch of Nazis were killed. Petros caught my eyes and waved his hand dismissively. "No great loss." Incensed, the Nazis told the Romanian soldiers to gather the Jews in the town and take them to the cemetery. Apparently, one of the gathered Jews noted a Jewish name on a headstone, and a woman started to wail as others chanted the religious prayer to honor God and the dead (it begins "Schma y'israel"). No doubt the sound was alien to the surrounding soldiers, yet to the Jews, it was spiritual and atavistic, bringing them in touch with their ancestors. Head bent, with halting speech, Petros told me that in the midst of the wailing, he heard a pop, then many pops; gradually he realized the sounds were gunfire. "I don't know who started it," he whispered. "This was not an order I gave, yet I feel terrible about it." Here he paused as it was an effort for him to continue. "All of them—all of the Jews, women, children, old men—were gunned down." All in all, he thought the total was more than ten thousand.

His eyes welled with tears as he said, "Some of my best friends are Jewish," and added, "everyone knows about my Jewish friends." He acknowledged that he was the commander, but it seemed to him that he lost his command for a moment. "No need for my family to know," he said. "No one else knows. Still I am sorry. I would like to apologize."

An hour had passed, and as we sat across each other, I wondered whether he knew that he would one day find a Jew to say this to. Can one slide out of guilt by an act of contrition? Did he look to me for repentance and salvation? I was not outraged or horrified. Here was someone directly associated with the killings that I had always heard about and regarded with disgust and fury, yet my only reaction was one of shock. Or perhaps, when the action is comprehensible, outrage comes as easy as it does when we are cut off in traffic; incomprehensible behavior overwhelms.

And we said good-bye. The stitches had been removed, and the wound was healing, leaving only a small jagged scar.

THE MAN WHO MET HITLER AND EINSTEIN

Lying on his deathbed, Hans H. appeared nothing like the powerful Austrian Nazi he once was. At age seventy-seven, he was riddled with malignant tumors that extended through the wall of his lower intestine, invading his urinary tract. Bowel and urine contaminants were leaking into his body. Cancer and infection were killing him, and the treatments weren't doing much to make his situation any better. He knew he was dying and accepted the fact with a calm resignation. Perhaps for that reason, he was eager to tell his story.

"I did not pick to become a Nazi," he said. "When Hitler moved into Austria, the male population of the country was suddenly obligated to serve in the German armed forces, and there I was in the Nazi army when I was about twenty." Because of his background in physics, he became a radio navigator in the German air force, which he told me was extremely dangerous because it involved high numbers of combat missions resulting in frequent casualties. His squadron flew sorties at the Russian front, where they bombed and strafed specific targets. In general, out of every three sorties, two planes would not go back. The survival statistic was about 30 percent, but Hans believed that statistics didn't mean a thing: the probability of each new event is independent of the previous event. He flew fifty-seven missions. In six of those missions, he was the only survivor.

He knew about concentration camps but denied knowledge of the Holocaust and even claimed a lack of sympathy with the German cause. While in Austria, he developed negative opinions about the "brown side—Nazis filled with arrogance" and the "black side—Catholic clergy who would abuse their power and make concessions to the Nazis in order to maintain their lifestyle of corruption while the scent of incense created the smell of religion." He said that he appreciated the quote of a fellow physicist, Professor Steven Weinberg, who once said, "With or without religion good people will do good things and evil people will do evil things, but it takes religion to get good people to do evil things."

Seated across from me that day, he told me, "The priests insisted upon fanatical religious belief, yet many of these same priests were known to abuse altar boys. The sacred masks the profane." Thus, he did not feel as much an anti-Nazi sentiment as he felt angered and disturbed by the whole system of abuse and hypocrisy. The Catholic Church worked with Hitler in order to keep their own dictatorial power, even to the extent of developing their own concentration camps (primarily for left-wingers and some Jews). He made reference to Nazi persecutions and exterminations, which were perpetrated by ordinary people formulated by a regime, an ideology, and a political culture. He returned to the realm of statistics when he mentioned that he was struck by the quote (misattributed to Stalin) "The death of one man is a tragedy, the death of a million is a statistic."

Somehow, Hans was able to keep his feelings to himself and, after his fifty-seventh mission, was moved to the Physics Institute in Berlin, where he worked on new weapons systems for the Nazis. It was there that he met Max Planck (who developed the basis for quantum theory) and Werner Heisenberg (who won the Nobel Prize for his work on quantum mechanics and developed the uncertainty principle of physics). During this period, Hans was introduced to Hitler but found him ignorant and arrogant, unable to truly appreciate physics. Hans published some important scientific papers, and after the war, he was listed as one of several promising scientists that the United States rushed to pick up before the Russians could find them. The Americans considered Hans among their top catches. The US government moved his family, their dog, and seven thousand pounds of furniture to the United States.

Soon after, Hans was working on photoelectric emissions. Eyes ablaze, and with his speech punctuated by coughing jags, he told me, "I provided the first spectrally resolved intensity measurements of radiation from the sun below 1,200 angstroms. This resulted in freeing electrons, which disassociates oxygen to develop the ozone layer." (It is that layer that provides a degree of protection from the sun's rays.) It was because of his work in the field that he met Albert Einstein, who shared an interest in photoelectric effects (for which he had been awarded the Nobel Prize in Physics).

As he lay dying, Hans spoke of his faith in democracy, which he described as "an almost violent belief." His certainty included his concept of evolution of the human species, which he stated was to replace the strongest with the wisest. He was proud of his membership in a "club of highly educated people in very high positions, breaking through academia and the media—*ubermenschen*." He felt this club would choose wise leaders and would make the proper decisions to direct the world. I wanted to ask him if this wasn't a bit too similar to the arguments made on behalf of a "super race," but he was too ill to continue the conversation that day. He died before we could resume our discussion.

I admired Hans's bravery and charm. His brilliance shined so brightly as to blind one to clouded moral and ethical issues, and I wondered whether I should have encouraged him to look beyond the bombing and the physics. A moment to speak out might have been possible; couldn't he express outrage or say no? What troubled me was the ease with which he could accept positions of a mercenary. He was aware of the hypocrisy and brutality that constituted the Nazi regime, yet he chose to cooperate and not speak out. That, along with his undying concept of a master race, made for a disturbing visit with a former Nazi on his way to his death.

He was my patient and I treated him for his medical problems, and I appreciated the opportunity to have our conversations. Yet I was also troubled with the realization that this permitted me to put a human face on a Nazi.

A physician must maintain a professional distance and remain objective in order to render the best possible care. However, when all is said and done, the moral ambiguity remains. I can't get even with Nazis. Their damage has been done.

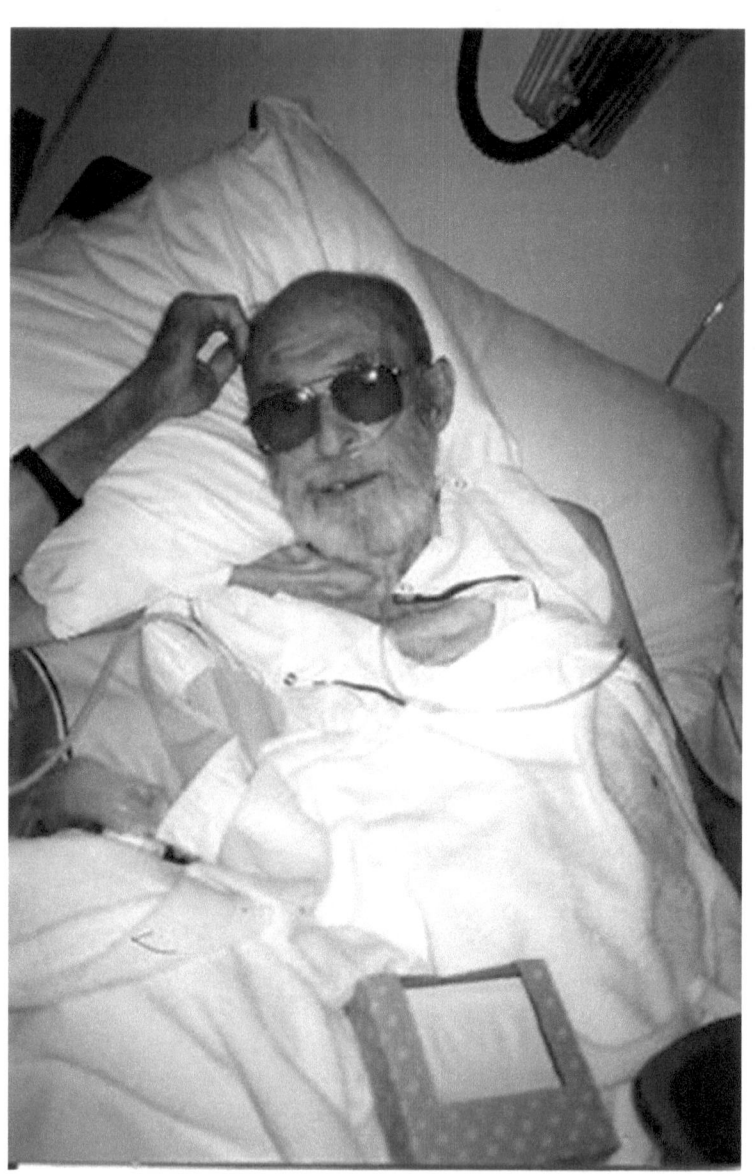

During the course of history there are points of transition; I've mentioned a few throughout this book. These occur as moments of decision, perhaps an opportunity to make an alternative choice whereby the result is different, following along the path set forth by a moral compass that leads to something better. We tend to push aside that choice in order to be less disruptive, afraid to be divisive. And that's when we fail to do what we know is right.

INSPIRATION

When I first met Jan B. in 1984, he was stooped, wheezy, with chaotic wisps of gray hair covering his aging scalp. His German accent was similar to countless others who had emigrated from Europe to America after World War II. His manner of speech was peppered with his sarcastic wit. Although he arranged the appointment at my office for an initial medical visit, pulling information from him was like yanking a resistant root from a long neglected garden. But eventually, the root was extricated and with it a rich soil of information.

Breathing was a problem for him. He had smoked for many years; the smoking began in Germany during difficult years, including war years, years when family was lost, years of imprisonment and exile, and years of progressive dyspnea. During that time, he wrote. His writings were often prophetic and politically important, and his writings got him into trouble. Because of the importance of his writing, he felt a burden to get each word right. Each word was timed with a drag from his omnipresent cigarette.

His father was a brick mason, a very good one according to Jan, who wanted advanced education for his son and encouraged him to go to college in Freiburg, Germany. He cautioned Jan that it is easy to sell one's soul, but resale value is prohibitive, thus impressing an ethic upon his young son. Jan acceded to his father's wishes in 1936 and then, out of curiosity, transferred to another school in East Prussia in 1937. There he worked on a newspaper with fellow students penning political tracts with increasingly pointed attacks against the regime.

The mood in the country seemed to be one of bewildered acquiescence, and Jan felt more like a reluctant witness to the range of horror that was unfolding. He felt as though he had been spending years in the anteroom, waiting for life to begin. Awaiting a brilliant, more meaningful existence, yet not quite knowing what exactly it was he was waiting for, he simply went ahead with his life. He supposed that once or twice in a lifetime you have those moments when you see or hear something that tilts your life just slightly in another direction, and only in retrospect, Jan appreciated that his life tilted against windmills, like that of Don Quixote.

Although Jan was not Jewish, he would occasionally write about the plight of the Jews (there was a lot to write about in those days). In 1940 he became part of the Resistance, writing and publishing anti-Nazi material, attempting to expose lies and corruption. To hear him tell it, he was no hero. He was not particularly drawn to the Resistance (he was never truly drawn to anything and never fashioned himself a joiner). It was the many things he opposed that drove him to write. His writings on the Nazis were like Cassandra's prophecies: speaking truth to unbelieving audiences. He had a special sense of injustice; he couldn't tell me why, but he seemed to readily see through propaganda. He had the ability to artfully articulate his beliefs, and it was his writing that endeared him to the Resistance. After finishing a piece, he dropped it off at an appointed place, and somebody picked it up and distributed it. To protect the organization and one another, those involved never crossed paths.

This worked until his sister, married to a Nazi functionary, turned him in. He was sent first to Dachau and then Auschwitz, but it was his role as a "political prisoner" that got him sent to a different eastern European concentration camp. The Nazis kept trying to find his collaborators: Who were the others? Where did he get his materials? Who were the printers and the writers? However, he was unable to be identified, and he couldn't identify others. He told me, "My captors had made a mistake. Like so many in the Resistance, I had grown a beard. When I was interned, the guards cut my hair and shaved my beard. The food was lousy, and treatment was subhuman. My weight dropped from 160 to 86, and no one could recognize me."

"Some prisoners would crack," he said. "They would run out and grab hold of a forty-thousand-volt wire surrounding the camp, thus committing suicide. People would be shot for nothing. Guards would call roll in the morning and, out of every fifth or tenth, or whatever the figure was, would take them out and shoot them for no apparent reason." But Jan felt that the worst part was that people lost faith and hope. In the meantime, he bartered for cigarettes and writing material. Although on occasion he successfully accumulated enough to write with, none of his writings from then survived.

The prisoners were soon to be liberated by two allied weapons carriers manned by Americans and Canadians. However, the Nazis knew that the liberators were coming, and the last day before liberation, they turned the machine guns from the watchtowers into the camp and shot as many people as they could. The barracks were made of thin planks of wood and were incapable of stopping bullets; splinters of wood flew as bullets popped through those thin walls to hit their unfortunate targets. Jan was one of the few survivors.

After the war, as Soviet power expanded, he traveled to eastern Europe and was involved in writing anti-Communist tracts, angering the establishment, which was also now developing a reputation for killing or imprisoning critics of the regime. He was thus forced into exile. He had experienced the despair of imprisonment and then the futility of exile. That was the punishment for writing down his ideas and beliefs; he missed the sights, the smells and the language of his youth, yet he kept on writing as if he were filled with youthful energy. His smoking continued as well—through the ambivalence of the loss of the sister who turned him over to the Nazis, the sudden death of his wife, and finally, the cancer death of his only child. Then the writing stopped, and only the smoking remained. He was reminded of the Tolstoy quote, "Happy people have no history."

When I met him, he was having trouble catching his breath. He spoke as a dampness formed in his wrinkled eye sockets, and he had developed a blue tinge to his lips due to depleted oxygen in his bloodstream. He said that asking the bigger questions only led to despair, and he even had trouble drawing the simplest of breaths: inspiration.

CAMP

"I can't tolerate it when people stand around at parties and talk about the camp they went to when they were children," H. B. blurted that out in her harsh Dutch accent as she overheard my conversation in the hospital corridor. I had arranged to have her plugged coronary arteries bypassed a week earlier, and now pus was leaking from the site of the surgical scar due to a postoperative infection. I needed to sign her case out to a colleague for the weekend because I was driving to Maine in order to take one of my children to camp.

H. B.'s family, a Jewish tribe that left Portugal in the 1400s, moved to Holland to escape the Inquisition. She was eleven when the Germans entered Holland on May 9, 1940, bombing Rotterdam in the dead of night. She remarked how Jews were killed, and non-Jews were dying by the thousands in an attempt to save Jews. The Germans would find a Jewish family hidden in a Christian home, take out all the Jews, and ship them to camps. The Christians were shot on the spot.

In February 1941, the entire Dutch railroad went on strike. From the president to the lowest level, they would not cooperate with the Germans. The Germans became vengeful; they wanted the railroad people more than they wanted the Jews. Many of the Dutch were harmed, but not one of them broke and no one returned to work until

1946. This was in distinct contrast to Poland, where people cheered by the roadside as Jews passed on their way to the camps.

In Israel today, there is a place overlooking Jerusalem called Yad Vashem, where a memorial stands to honor martyrs and heroes of the Holocaust. The man who tried to save H. B. is honored there on the Street of the Righteous Gentile. He was Catholic, one of the local boys friendly with H. B. and her brother. Two of those boys imitated their parents, enlisting their friends to help them save hundreds of Jewish children. "There was a courtyard in my town where thousands of Jews had been gathered," H. B. said. "The boys killed two German soldiers and put on their uniforms. One of them entered the courtyard, and one remained at the wall outside. The one who entered tried to convince the mothers of small children and babies that he was trying to help. They knew the mothers would not survive, but tried to save the children." The boy would take the child from its mother and yell, "This little Jew thing, I'm going to kill it," and toss it over the wall to his brother, who, in turn, would take it to the nuns to hide. One of the boys was caught and shot. The other escaped and remained within the network of resistance fighters.

H. B. had been in hiding on her own, but a man who was supposed to protect her tried to rape her. Using the complex underground network, she contacted her friend (one of the surviving boys), who managed to find her and take her to where her father and brother were hiding. They were able to hide there for two years until someone turned them in for the reward of one hundred guilders a head. They were taken to a prison called the Hell of Holland, and then, if they survived, they were to be sent to Westerbork concentration camp.

In the jail, soldiers beat her father and stole a watch and a gold pencil set from him. They sold the pilfered items, which allowed them to go out and party. The prisoners were left for two days with no toilet and nothing to eat. The stench was awful and filled their senses, but smells were the least of their problems. When the soldiers returned pie-eyed, they hauled the Jews out and loaded them in cars to take them to the camp. Halfway out of town, they stopped and lined the prisoners up in a ditch. H. B.'s father put his arms around his son and daughter and said, "You must have courage. I don't want you to cry or carry on. The sons of bitches are going to kill us. Don't give in."

"It was a beautiful speech," H. B. told me. Yet her family was not shot. By chance, the soldiers had been so drunk that they'd forgotten bullets. H. B. and her family were shoved back into the cars and continued to their destination: camp. She recalled the ride was pretty quiet, punctuated only by guffaws from the soldiers and the sound of her father weeping. The hours they spent together had more value than diamonds.

When H. B. arrived at the camp at Westerbork, the Nazi guards cut her hair with a knife and placed her in work barracks. There she witnessed soldiers tossing infants in the air in order to compete to see who could kill it with the fewest shots fired. She saw lots of death, but the first time she witnessed a noncontorted death was when her dog died. She found it particularly moving that the death of an animal was more peaceful than that of a child.

H. B. grew up without thinking of herself as Jewish in spite of the intense reminder of her background. However, she recognized the Jewish memorial prayer for the dead at a friend's funeral she attended as an adult. The prayer begins, "Yis gadol v yis gadash," and at that funeral, she turned to her husband and said, "I know that prayer, because in the camp, people said it for themselves since they knew no one would be able to say it for them." She told me that there was another prayer they said, "Schma yisreal adonai elohanu adonai echad." Heard from the gas chambers, it was chanted in camp—a very different camp song.

THE ROLE OF WRITING

In the course of talking to my patients, I developed the sense that listening and recording these stories were somehow helping my patients heal in a more subtle way. Of course, that may not be true, but it's hard to quibble since with each telling, there appears to be a feeling of gratitude and catharsis expressed by the patient. If I can get the stories down, the story is preserved, the patient is remembered, the story is kept, then it's done. We are not complete without a narrative. Time and again, my patients will present to the office or the hospital with a malady, but they want me to get a picture of who they are; they want me to understand their story. Maybe, in addition to the chance for cure, I represent a safe haven for them.

Michael W. was only forty-eight, and I was concerned about the discomfort he felt in his chest. Not unexpectedly, it proved to be a heart attack. Yet when the disease was successfully treated, the malady remained. It was, I eventually realized, a story waiting to be released.

Michael was born in Germany shortly after World War II but moved to Boston when he was still a young man. His mother was German and had been a member of Nazi youth; his father was an American soldier stationed in Germany. He felt a lot was ignored after the war. In his words, things were "swept under the carpet, and we pretend it never happened." In his view, this was not done out of shame; he knew there were people who believe it's terrible that the Germans lost. He noted two schools of thought: those who, to this day, would probably follow another Hitler, if there was one, concentration camps and all; and those like his family, who kept a lid on the whole question.

The reason Michael's family doesn't discuss the Nazis is that his father was half Jewish. Anti-Semitism was inescapable in Germany, and Michael discovered it within his own family. He recalled the night when his parents called him into a room to tell him, in hushed tones, that his grandfather was Jewish. The Jewish blood was on his father's side, those still living in Chicago. His Jewish grandfather had married an Irish Catholic girl and was ostracized by his family. After his grandfather died, his grandmother raised his father as a Catholic.

Since Michael was born to an American parent on official business, he was granted automatic American citizenship with the stipulation that he return to the United States every six years or lose citizenship. He first came to Chicago as a child, a few years after the end of the war. The irony is that he had a Jewish surname and was living in a Jewish neighborhood, and other children in that Chicago neighborhood threw bricks at him because he was blond and could only speak German. They all thought he was a little Nazi. In first grade, he had to fight his way to and from school. Nobody even asked him whether he was American, German, Jewish, Protestant, or Catholic. At age six, he went to a Catholic parochial school in Chicago's west side and was attacked because they thought he was a Nazi, but he didn't know what a Nazi was.

As we spoke, his eyes darted around my office as if looking for an explanation, "I don't think too many six-year-olds know what a Nazi is." Michael didn't feel that prejudice only happened through ignorance and misunderstanding. He felt it also began with personal unhappiness. He told me, "Once you feel bad about yourself, you can feel bad about anybody. You start picking on little things or big things—it doesn't matter what it is—but by bringing the other person down, you bring yourself up. Thinking back on it now, I'm sure I can understand where those kids who attacked me in Chicago were coming from. This was just after the war. There had been all this terrible tragedy, and obviously my brother Tom (in kindergarten) and I were considered to be the enemy who had just landed in the neighborhood. But I have to say that nobody stopped to ask us who we were before they attacked us. We were Americans, and we certainly weren't Nazis. But, you know, nobody asked."

At one point, Michael's father attempted to empathize with his children and described his own experience with prejudice. Michael was ambivalent about his father because of the Jewish roots and the forced move to the neighborhood in Chicago, which put him in this complicated position in the first place. His father was raised Catholic, in a mostly Protestant neighborhood, and he recalled being taunted as a "cat-licker" when he went to school. When Michael was a child, he didn't know why his father was telling him about this, but as Michael was relating his story to me, his eyes filled with softness and sorrow as he said he now realized that his father was attempting to relate to his son's situation. Michael's father told him that taunting with the term "cat-licker" was meant to be derogatory, but his father was a child and couldn't understand why, only that it was a perversion of the word Catholic. "There is so much that a child does not understand. They called them cat-lickers in those days," Michael said. "People would say you were 'nothing but a cat-licker.'"

As Michael recalled this, he said that he finally understood what his father was trying to explain to him; the emotional pain seemed to subside. The pressure in his chest was gone, the heart attack was treated with medication, and then he underwent successful cardiac catheterization with placement of a stent that opened up his plugged coronary artery. Michael felt that "you must reflect on the past in order to move forward, but sometimes you can't, and you move backward."

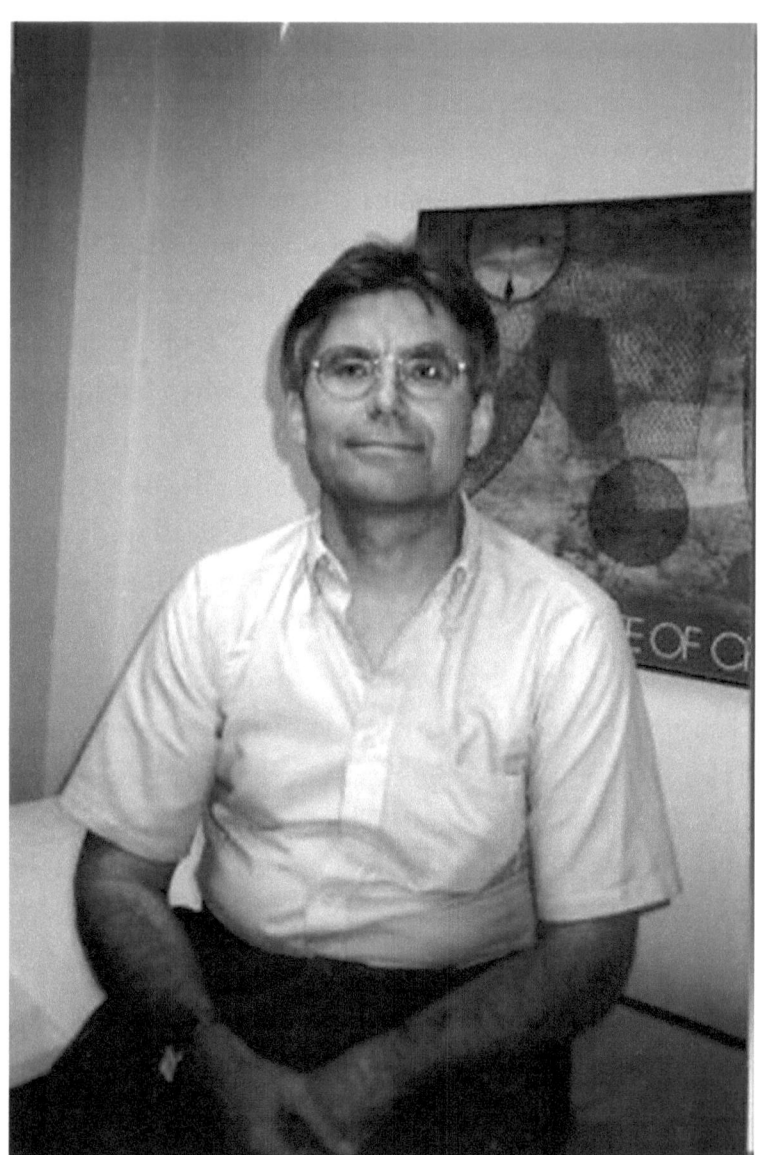

ALLIANCES

World War II engendered strict alliances. Primarily, it was us (America, Britain, Russia) against them (Germany, Japan, Italy) with smaller countries taking sides as the conflict progressed. Lee Mazuto's family, living in California, was well aware of those alliances, and they came down firmly on the side of America and its allies. His family moved from Japan to California in the 1930s when Lee was only six. I met him more than fifty years later, an elderly man who retained the stooped reverential posture and thick Japanese accent of his parents. His manner was gentle, and he exuded beneficence and kindness. He recalled for me that his parents established a small business; they were disciplined, serious, and hardworking. "When I came home from school after doing well on a test," he told me, "the first question my mother would ask was, 'Ninety-five is a good grade, but did anybody get one hundred?'" He and his family believed in the "American way"—the way of the allies.

Then, on a clear December day in 1941, Japan bombed Pearl Harbor. America was soon at war, and the nation was mobilized. As this country shifted to a wartime mentality, the population took on a patriotic fervor, which Lee and his family briefly shared. However, they were not actually accepted as mainstream Americans. Earl Warren, the attorney general at that time, made a point of saying that America should expect sabotage from the Japanese within the country. Perversely, Americans came to believe that the longer the wait without an attack, the more likely an attack would be. As the fear grew, so did anti-Japanese sentiment, including fear of Japanese Americans. The word went out that "hiring a Jap is an insult to patriotic Americans," and William Randolph Hearst (owner of Hearst Newspapers) opined that "the only good Jap is a dead Jap." The Chinese walked around with badges saying, "I'm not Japanese." In February 1942, President Roosevelt signed orders setting up camps to "relocate" Japanese living in the United States. Although Germans and Italians were monitored as well, it was the Japanese who were evacuated.

In April 1942, Lee and his family were told to leave their home and enter an internment camp, just like 120,000 other Japanese Americans. At that time, Lee's older brother was in the US Army, and his mother was convinced her family was from samurai ancestry and, thus, believed in the samurai code. She said to her son, "If you have to fight and if you have to die, die with dignity." The family retained support for America and its allies, despite their circumstances. They cooperated with the evacuation.

They never saw their books and furniture again, but Lee was only thirteen and thought this could be fun. Books and furniture seemed a small price to pay for the freedom of two extra months out of school. Eventually, the family was transported to Topaz, Utah, where they were housed in large barracks made of pine wood with tar paper siding—eight people for two rooms. The camp was surrounded by barbed wire. All around the perimeter were attack dogs and armed guards who could shoot them if they attempted to escape. His infant nephew had pneumonia, but there was no medicine and no hospital. The camp was very dusty, and relatives determined that the baby must have had allergies, which contributed to his death.

"The dust was like flour powder," Lee said. "You slept with it, ate it, you breathed it. The people covered with fine powder gave the macabre appearance of ghosts passing." When Lee came to see me, he was suffering from severe pulmonary disease without a clear source except for those early exposures, which I explained was similar to smoking thousands of cigarettes.

The feeling in the camp was that life was completely disrupted. Yet for the youngsters, this was all right. It was a break in the life of a traditional Japanese family, an environment where parents had a firm grip on the children. Now youngsters, like Lee and his allies, were on their own. Lee remembered the tears and the shame of his mother as she tried to cope with the many humiliations, having departed from the once proud and disciplined Japanese tradition. He bowed his head as he recalled the dark circles under her eyes, which provided a stark, maybe cruel, contrast to the bright blue cloudless sky that seemed to mock their existence.

In October 1945 the government decided the camps weren't cost-efficient, and they released the interned Japanese. Lee's family didn't know where to go but decided on Cincinnati, Ohio, because it was rumored there was a little less prejudice against the Japanese in that area. They were an oddity, though. Ohioans hadn't heard much about the camps, and they didn't seem interested to hear about them, which provoked, in Lee, great confusion and grief. He was able to leave Ohio and attend college in Boston, where he became an engineer. He remained in the Boston area to raise his family.

There exists a virus that causes a painful inflammation and a blistering rash when it invades the nerves. This virus, herpes zoster, or shingles, is closely associated with the chickenpox virus, which lies dormant in the nerve ganglion for many years after the initial bout of chickenpox. Some physicians believe the virus flares up for no reason, but others say great stress or immune problems lead to its emergence. I don't know why Lee developed a severe case of herpes zoster, but I do know that it occurred while he was planning a trip to show his two teenage daughters Topaz, Utah; painful vesicles began rising like the Phoenix from ash. The nerve pain lasted throughout the trip.

Lee Mazuto's story about the United States' internment of Japanese during World War II reminds me of the novel by the Nobel laureate author J. M. Coetzee *Waiting for the Barbarians*. The novel is about a small village, an island of civility, in an undescribed time and place. The inhabitants are kind and generous until the day a rumor spreads that barbarians are on the way to destroy the village. As the villagers prepare for the arrival of the barbarians, the once-civilized people become less civilized and more barbaric. By the time it is determined that there are no barbarians on the way, the people of the village have become the barbarians themselves.

THURSDAY — **San Francisco Examiner Editorial Page** — MAY 6, 1943

For U.S. Safety • Keep Japs in Internment

THE recent hullabaloo by naive sentimentalists, demanding the release of Jap civilians from relocation centers under one pretext or another, has aroused the resentment and apprehension of the Pacific coast.

The plain fact is that the Government in Washington hardly seems to consider the west coast as part of the United States, and cares little about what might happen to us here.

The Government has learned nothing from Pearl Harbor, nor has it any intelligent realization of the importance of the Pacific war.

The agitation over the Jap internees is a natural consequence of this sort of thinking, or rather lack of thinking.

To Washington, the question seems remote and academic.

But to us on the Pacific coast, the matter is of the most immediate concern.

District Attorney Fred N. Howser of Los Angeles County spoke to the point when he said:

"I know Japs as well as the average Caucasian, but I would never accept the serious job of deciding which Japs to release and which to keep under surveillance. There is no one I know with sufficient wisdom to make this selection with safety. The proponents of liberating Japs overlook the fact that we are engaged in a war in which the stakes are the lives of our families and ourselves....

"I say regardless of any imaginary injustice being done a few, that the welfare of the whole Nation makes it mandatory that we never relax our vigilance over interned Japanese."

That is well put, logical and sensible.

It boils down to this: That there is no judicial or scientific method of determining a Jap's loyalty or harmlessness, and that to waste time and effort to attempt the test, would be distracting attention from the war effort and adding to the general concern over the Nation's internal safety.

As Mr. Howser puts it:

"We have no time or desire to keep a close watch on released Japs, who at present are safe in relocation centers, where sabotage, communication with the enemy and subversive activities are impossible."

So let's get on with the work of survival and victory and hope that no further nonsense of this type comes from Washington to plague us.

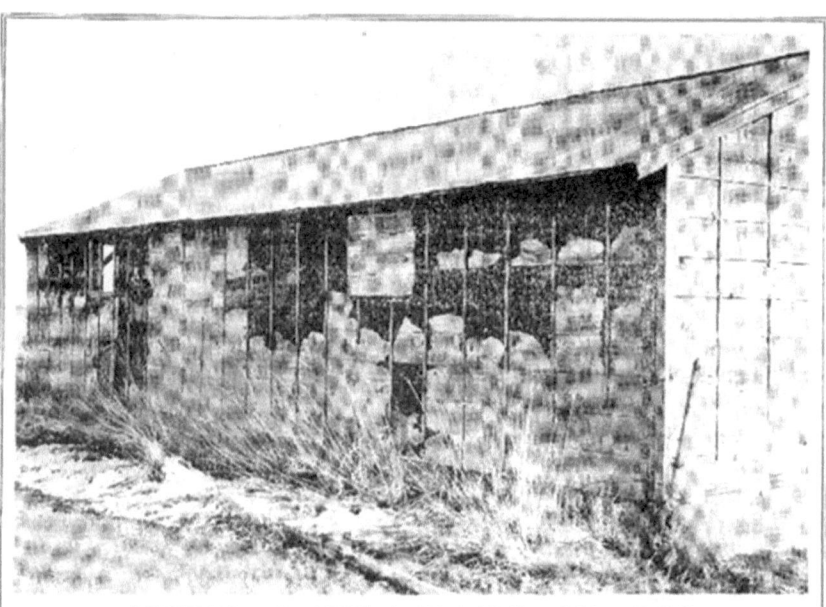

Lingering remains of the tar paper siding reveals that this former's barn was once a Topaz barrack. The original buildings were cut into pieces before they were moved from the site. When the camp first opened, some of the structures were not yet completed even though Japanese Americans were assigned to these barracks. Some did not have sheet rock in the interiors. None had insulation except for the tar paper siding. The first contingent arrived from Tanforan around September 16, 1942. By September 19, Delta's temperature fell to 29. The morning was clear weather with a north wind bringing frost.

December 1982

TRUTH—JUSTICE   San Francisco Examiner Editorial Page

Ickes' Hiring of Japs on Farm Is Insult to Patriotic Americans

HAROLD ICKES, Secretary of the Interior, has astounded Americans by removing from relocation centers in the West individual Japanese to work on his private farm.

This is the same Mr. Ickes who has just written "The Autobiography of a Curmudgeon." This book is as cheap a performance of self-confessional exhibitionism as we have ever had from a high ranking Government official in our history.

His employment of Japs that his own Government have interned may be either part of this element in his character of defiant and nauseating public exhibitionism or, it may be part of the Administration's seemingly general disregard of the Japanese menace.

Whatever Mr. Ickes' motive for thus defying the patriotic and protective sentiment of the country HIS DEVOTION NOW SEEMS CLEARLY TO BE ONLY TO THAT PART OF THE COUNTRY WHICH HE PERSONALLY OWNS.

The Pacific League, over the signatures of Russ Avery, president of the League, and Frederic T. Woolman, chairman of the League's alien problems committee, has taken Curmudgeon Ickes to task in a vigorous letter sent direct to the Secretary.

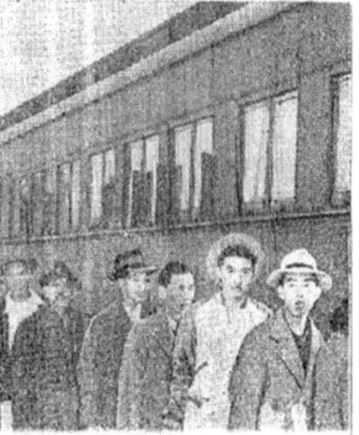

TREACHERY, LOYA
INHERENT JA

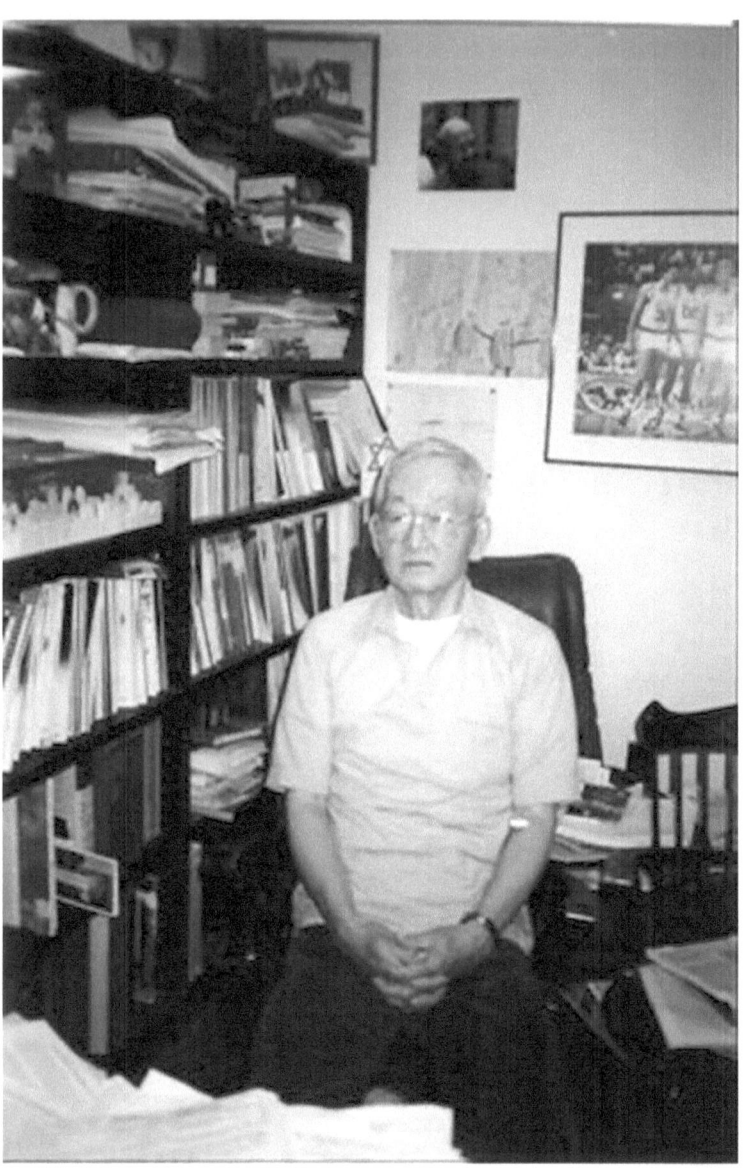

    I guess there is such a thing as junk,
I've heard about it,
    read about it,
pondered its existence,
    but have never seen it;
no rusted-out vehicle, dilapidated couch,
        worn-out shirt, torn underwear,
perforated stamp, ripped envelope,
        stained carpet, broken wristwatch,
legless table, chipped cup,
        cracked plate, sunken mattress,
backless chair,
    shattered, disheveled old man
is without a story
    there is no junk

POETRY

She would smile and almost bounce into the office with the confidence of a patient with no fears. This contrasted with my worldview that the sky was falling and I was the early witness. Perhaps I could appreciate her effervescence and understand her ability to remain cheerfully philosophical about whatever comes her way.

"We need to study history in order to produce poetry, a necessity of all human civilizations. By knowing history, I can seek out beauty. Also, it is the poets who describe most vividly how man fell," Thelma V. explained to me as we sat across each other following a routine physical exam. Because of the discovery of some abnormal lab tests, she had spent most of the day going from my office to the X-ray department at the adjoining hospital and back to my office to discuss the results. The day was spent with her going back and forth while I continued to see a constant stream of patients.

It was now early evening as she relaxed in her chair in my office. She was seated across me, and her face had a rosy glow as she peered at the setting sun through the window behind my back. She appeared younger than her sixty-eight years. Her breast prostheses gave a casual observer no indication of the bilateral mastectomies. As we chatted, she told me she had wanted to write her memoirs but had wound up writing poems instead.

For years Thelma V. had been taking estrogen hormone therapy to reduce her menopause symptoms. Breast tissue has estrogen receptors, which utilize the hormone to stimulate tissue function. This process can increase DNA replication, including duplication of a mutated or changed DNA strand if one exists. Cancer can result from the continued reproduction of the changed DNA. This means that the stimulus from estrogen can, unknowingly to the patient, increase the production of a mutant cell. About a third of patients with breast cancer have an inherited predisposition to the disease, which implies that they have a greater chance than the rest of the population of having a cancer-causing mutation in their DNA. Thelma had a strong family history of breast cancer, making the use of estrogen that much less advisable.

But in those days, almost thirty years ago when it was prescribed to her, the estrogen risk was not as well established as it is now. Studies were contradictory, and doctors felt that helping women cope with menopause was compassionate. She asked, "What makes a charlatan a charlatan and not simply a believer in false prophets?" It may be fake knowledge, but perhaps, for the most naive, it is science without skepticism.

Thelma noticed she had a breast lump and brought it to the attention of her only doctor at that time, her gynecologist. He asserted that the estrogen he had been prescribing for a decade could not have had a deleterious effect on her breast tissue. The lump had developed after several years of estrogen hormone stimulus and was ultimately proved to be a cancer. The treatment offered was a mastectomy, repeated on the remaining breast when recurrence was noted a few years later. My job, on the day we discussed poetry, was to review her treatment with estrogen-blocking agents and look for evidence of treatment side effects or cancer spread and discuss treatment of her arthritic joints as well as to evaluate her general health.

"I've survived worse," she told me of her experience with cancer. "This just gets added to my life's tapestry." (The way a patient tells their story has given me a sense of how they will deal with whatever news I have to give them. This is true of all the doctor-patient interactions I've included, and it creates bilateral trust as difficult diagnosis and treatment occur.) Heartened by her attitude, I told her that her test results weren't all normal. "Your liver enzymes are elevated. It may not be serious, but I want to arrange a liver scan for today and will discuss those results with you afterwards." She fluffed her hair and stared out the window for about a minute. My secretary was able to arrange for the scan that day, and I asked Thelma to see me to discuss the results after the scan was completed a few hours later. The scan came back normal, and I determined the enzyme abnormality was due to an effect of her anti-inflammatory medications used to treat arthritis. She replied that she would have been able to handle whatever the results. As she looked me in the eye, she said, "My generation already experienced fear and struggle, so I've had practice dealing with difficult situations. I can accept what comes my way."

However, she worried about her two grown daughters' cancer risk and their inability to cope with life struggles. She felt that they could not deal with the concept of "fate," whether it arose from what was programmed into their genes or from whatever form it seeped into their lives. "When I try to talk to my daughters," she said, "they think I am telling stories. But I tell them anyway. They need to know." She settled into her chair across my paper-strewn desk. Although she had arrived in my office in the morning, by the time we were able to go over her test results, it was early evening. My patient visits for the day were complete, with the exception of Thelma, and she related her story to me:

> World War II was long ago, but it stays with you a long time. We were without anything and had just come out of an economic

depression when the war began. During the stock market crash of 1929, two men, who had lost everything, committed suicide by jumping off a bridge in the path of a train. My father knew them and hoped he could avoid their fate by maintaining his little fruit stand that he built when he emigrated here from Albania. Fortunately, he had some success and was able to build a store.

Thelma's chubby face and high cheekbones gave her a look of permanent merriment, yet her face grew dark as she continued.

One day as I left the store, I saw a dead body in the parking lot. It was a man who had shot himself because he could no longer feed his family. As a child living in the midst of a confusing time, I feared for the survival of my own father because he was earning less than the family needed. He tried to hide his problems, which only magnified the fear.

But this country moved forward, Thelma told me as I noticed the sky outside my window darken. The economy recovered a bit, some began to prosper, and Thelma's family survived.

I thought that might be the end of the story—a happy conclusion to difficult times—but Thelma continued, "We had closed our eyes and our ears to what was going on in Europe. We were a country that was fairly new, and we were just beginning to come out of this depression." Like many people, Thelma heard about the atrocities occurring in Europe but chose not to believe them. "We were an island unto ourselves," she told me. She heard tales of a madman in Germany but knew dictatorships were everywhere. People said that those affected by the problem should be the ones to deal with it. The situation seemed to have nothing to do with America, at least until Japan bombed Pearl Harbor.

"The reason that we ultimately got into the war was Japan—Pearl Harbor. Until that moment, December 7, around four o'clock in the afternoon, it was not real," Thelma told me. Her family listened to the radio constantly in those days. "It came over the radio, and we sat and listened. Sunday night was *Jack Benny* and *The Green Hornet*. At four o'clock, *Ellery Queen* had just ended and *Gang Busters* came on, and it was interrupted with the report that Pearl Harbor had been bombed." Even then, at thirteen, Thelma didn't know how the attack would impact her life. The events still seemed so far away.

"The next day in school, there was an assembly, and a teacher got up and said, 'You will never again live the life you have lived up until this moment.' He was right. Life changed immediately. Women hadn't worked outside the home but went into factories and took over men's jobs. Up to that moment, women were feminine, stayed at home, had the little crisp apron on, and did the cooking, just like the Walton family on TV. Mothers and wives said good-bye to their husbands. Children said good-bye to their fathers, many for the last time."

Transfixed by her account, I was gaining an understanding of my patient as well as the history and mood of the country I'd only read about in books. I encouraged Thelma to go on. "Despite being unprepared," she said, "the country mobilized quickly for war. People raised money for war bonds in order to support the war. Factories converted. Instead of cars, they made tanks. Steel became precious."

Americans had rules to follow, and like the rest of her countrymen, Thelma drew thick black curtains over the windows at night so that no lights would shine to give a plane a chance to see if it was a big city or something worth bombing.

She smoothed the lap of her skirt and had the look of someone caught deep within a once-forgotten memory as she murmured, "We were scared of an imminent attack. While atrocities were going on in

Europe, we were so busy fighting this war that it seemed insignificant. We were too busy fighting for ourselves, for our own existence." Thelma noted that life seemed surreal and wondered if it could return to normal.

"This country was unprepared for anything but picked itself up in a few months: boys enlisted, some too young, so they lied about their age in order to serve in the army; women joined the workforce; and we finally gave support to England and prevented a German victory. My sister's husband learned to kill and went over and fought in the Battle of the Bulge. His friends died or lost arms or legs. He came back looking whole yet seemed to have lost everything. Although they were fortunate they didn't need to put a gold star in their window, which indicated the loss of a husband or a son, maybe they should have. He was never the same upon his return, and my sister was never the same either."

Thelma's growing awareness of the suffering of others caused her to investigate the plight of family members who had remained in Albania. Many of them were starving; there wasn't even bread to eat. In 1939, Italy invaded Albania (Mussolini was an ally of Hitler). The Germans came next, isolating the town where Thelma's relatives lived, lining up townspeople and shooting them. "We saw it in the movies but didn't actually believe it," Thelma told me. "My first cousin was hidden by the French underground, which saved his life. That is why the Albanians welcomed the Communists at the end of the war: there finally was bread, and more importantly, they weren't living in terror."

I thought that Thelma had finished speaking. I sat thinking about her cancer risk, the fact that her bilateral mastectomies, though a missing part of her anatomy, had caused me to lose focus of the entire person, her experience with the Depression and World War II, and her ability to remember without bitterness. And as I rose to escort her to the door, she spoke.

"We are now left with our comfortable lives, trying to explain history and why we did what we did. With our powerful religious beliefs, we should have a covenant of responsibility, not privilege. That does not seem to be a popular message these days. I know this sounds corny, but we have to accept our fellowman, no matter what color or creed or what his thoughts are. He has the right to his own thoughts or belief and the freedom to view his own history and write his own poetry. I believe we need poetry with its views on despair and hope, from the *Iliad* through Dante's *Inferno* to *Leaves of Grass*. We need this, plus our internal poetic machinery, in order to understand our place in history."

Thelma is now considered a cancer survivor, but I'll keep an eye out for advancing disease, spread of tumor, areas of alarm, and the poetry of despair and hope.

MENTAL HEALTH

I believe in the merits of tensile strength, a property found in particular metals used in bridge and skyscraper foundations. That combination of flexibility plus hardness is crucial. We, of course, have a degree of that in our bones, the flexibility provided by a matrix of bridging fibers interspersed with fat, allowing the bone to bend but not break. However, it can break. Sometimes, when a long bone (such as the femur, in the upper leg) breaks, it releases chunks of fat that can shoot up through the veins to the lungs, resulting in respiratory failure. Thus, we all need a degree of tensile strength so that our bones don't just snap open.

Unfortunately for Philip, the long bones in his legs did snap when he was hit by a car as he walked out of a bar on New Year's Eve. The driver, with a suspended license, was drunk and left twenty-two-year-old Philip lying in the road with two broken femurs and a broken left humerus (all long bones with just enough tensile strength to handle only a certain degree of stress before they crack). Philip's mind was okay; in fact, on his third hospital day, he was mentally intact enough to notify the nursing staff that he felt more winded than usual. The medical staff determined that Philip's broken bones had released fat that shot up to his lungs; he would die unless the medical team could give him adequate oxygen. He was put on a membrane oxygenator called ECMO. In this system, catheters are placed in blood vessels, and the blood circulates through a machine, which mimics the lungs by removing carbon dioxide and replenishing oxygen, permitting the lungs to rest and repair. Because the procedure is complex, it is reserved for the direst cases.

Marsha, Philip's mother, was anxious about her son, but he wasn't her only problem. Two days prior to Philip's accident, Marsha had been sitting at dinner with her husband when he collapsed. He was taken to the hospital where he was fortunate enough to survive the subarachnoid hemorrhage (a brain bleed caused by a rupture of a ballooned-out cerebral artery). He remained in critical condition at a neighboring hospital. Marsha chose not to tell her husband about Philip's situation.

Marsha's other child, twenty-five-year-old Mark, had been trying to return from a snowed-in area ever since he had heard about his father. He was driving a rental car across the country, and when he called his mother to check in, she told him about his brother. Mark caught a flight the rest of the way home and has been living there ever since, supporting his mother. In response to the pressures of her husband's and son's medical problems, Marsha had become overwhelmed and withdrawn, so Mark was now making major family decisions.

A few years before, Mark had been struggling a bit through school, was in and out of minor jams, and was trying to figure out what to do with his life. Recently he had found his way and had been out on his own, securing an apartment and a good sales position. Things had been on the upswing until those final days of 2006. On the day he came to see me, he said he felt fine except for trouble swallowing and episodes of feeling like he couldn't breathe. I asked him if he felt the strain of his particular burden and wondered how it had affected his mental health. He said, "Don't worry about me. I'm as hard as steel!" I just hope that he has enough tensile strength.

Maybe it is adequate to be a sounding board or an outlet. Perhaps the doctor's office can provide a safe haven. I suspect that alone may be the reason why just listening can be therapeutic. Not all patients are willing to seek the help of a therapist.

THERAPY

"I find it therapeutic to pull out this picture in my wallet and think what could have been," Robert said when I suggested therapy to ease his stress and, perhaps, lower his blood pressure.

It was 1967, and he was twenty when he was summoned to Vietnam. He couldn't hack it in college, so enlisting seemed to be a reasonable alternative; after all, most of his friends were there. He joined them as a member of the infantry. He quickly discovered that the jungle was hot and unfriendly, and when it rained, you could not get dry. When he was frightened, he could not find relief. Most of the time, he was wet and scared.

But some of the guys seemed brave and managed to stay dry. How they did it, he never knew. They would sign up for repeat tours—always brave and always dry. The veterans took the new recruits under their wing. They always seemed to know more than their twenty-six-year-old lieutenant, who was way too enthusiastic and way too green. He tried to send the brave, dry guys out on dangerous missions to take a hill, lose some men, and retreat from the hill. Lieutenants and captains who did that too often would get fragged (injured or, possibly, killed by their own troops). Fragging became pretty common as the war wore on, and Robert's perky, enthusiastic lieutenant was fragged when a grenade was rolled under his cot.

Robert knew who tried to kill the lieutenant but wouldn't say. The army wouldn't jail him because they needed soldiers, and they wouldn't send him home because healthy soldiers weren't just sent home, so they "promoted" him to scout. His responsibility was to venture deep into the jungle and scout out the enemy. The dense bush crowded in with unnerving effect. Most scouts lasted less than two weeks. Alone in the deep jungle, Robert was terrified and lonely. His only company was the enemy.

One day he caught sight of a lone enemy soldier through the thick jungle vegetation, and just as their eyes met, registering surprise, fear, then resignation, he felt a sudden bond. He felt those frightened eyes mirrored his own and that they shared a fleeting common humanity. Nevertheless, his reaction was instinctive, and he shot off a round, killing the enemy soldier. Before he left the area, he took a picture of the boy he killed. "It was the only time I killed someone," he said. "I was never a gung-ho soldier, but I was in a desperate situation where I had to kill or be killed." He couldn't say that he had regrets about what he did. Still, he didn't feel quite right about it either.

Forty years later, he still carries the photo in his wallet. He does this out of respect for his victim, and he feels that in some way, it is therapeutic. He knows that his victim would have done the same for him; if circumstances had been reversed, the enemy soldier would remember Robert in some way. "I could tell this from the brief flash of fear and recognition, the look in his eyes," Robert said, "just before I shot."

Robert never developed a satisfactory relationship with a therapist, and his blood pressure is now well controlled with medication. We don't talk about Vietnam much anymore. He says that someday he would like to tell his kids about all this, but he's afraid that they'll never understand, so for now, he'll keep it to himself.

VULNERABILITY

Ray used to be a navy guy. That's where he got his tattoos. His broken nose came from a bar fight in Okinawa; he wasn't able to recall how the incisors disappeared. So when he presented to my office for a blood pressure check, I was alarmed to hear him say how shaken up he was.

He had just returned from a vacation in Greece, where he spent two glorious weeks with his second wife. As they were flying back on TWA Flight 847, a group of Islamic hijackers took over the plane. The hijackers shouted at the passengers, demanding they put their heads down between their knees, and if they rose, they would be shot. As the jihadists strolled down the aisles, they stopped to play Russian roulette with passengers. They drank whiskey and fondled the female flight attendants. Although they talked jihad, Ray could see their behavior did not mesh with Islamic code—he was sure this was not condoned in the Koran. "These guys were thugs with a veneer of a holy cause." When their demands weren't met, they shot and killed one of the passengers—a navy diver—and later tossed his dead body onto the tarmac. Ray turned to his wife and whispered, "We're dead meat."

Eventually, the plane returned to the Greek airport for refueling and to continue negotiations for hostage release. While there, Ray asked to go to the bathroom in order to put in eyedrops necessary to treat his glaucoma, which would cause blindness if left untreated. His wife was allowed to accompany him to the bathroom. Before they could return to their seats, they were taken, along with eight other hostages, and exchanged for prisoners (fellow jihadists) who had been previously captured and held at the Greek airport.

After Ray disembarked, he was able to put in the drops and could see again. One TV reporter commented on the news that a hostage faked his blindness to get off the plane. Hearing this, Ray became anxious and quite concerned for the safety of the remaining hostages. His blood pressure rose. (It was still high by the time I saw him.)

When he returned to the States, he related the story and asked me to contact the TV station to arrange a retraction. He felt that I could explain that he did not fake his medical condition. Because the crisis was ongoing, Ray seemed desperate. However, when I finally did reach the TV station, they informed me, "We can't verify that." And they kept the story as is. Eventually, the hostages were released. I'm not sure I can say the same for Ray. He kept his doubts about his experience bound deep within, only at times saying that he felt like a coward and could not seem to be convinced otherwise. How easy it is to steal someone's dignity!

TRANSITION

Stephen's eyes were wide-open with gleaming, dilated pupils as he entered my office. The abdominal pain, he said, was "like a hole is burning through, like a hole I can't fill." Additionally, he suffered from a six-month history of nausea, which had started just about the time he returned from Iraq. His voice was shaky, and his tattoos couldn't cover his fear; the transition back home had been exceedingly tough for him.

As a high school senior, Stephen signed up for the marines because he wasn't prepared for college and didn't know what else to do. He imagined how he would look to friends and family when he returned home from duty smartly dressed in his marine uniform. At age nineteen, he had just finished boot camp two weeks before the planes hit the World Trade Center towers on September 11, 2011. Later, when the United States decided to invade Iraq, Stephen's was among the first marine divisions to go. He did three tours: outside of Baghdad, Fallujah, and Ramadi. The enemy consisted of snipers, suicide bombers, and the omnipresent IEDs (improvised explosive devices).

The vehicles were not well equipped, and he was responsible for welding armor onto his Humvee. The doors had a tendency to flop open, and the soldiers had to hold them shut. Eight to ten soldiers loaded the back of the vehicles, and their heads rose over the top, making perfect targets for snipers. They viewed themselves as brothers, looking out for one another, no longer giving a thought to the rationale for this war, and trying to stay alive. The captain sat in the front, protected by four-inch glass windows. The enemy especially wanted to kill the captains as a particular prize and thus monitored all the soldiers' movements. "They watched us all the time," Stephen said. Videos were always taken, especially to capture the kills and maiming on film, in order to publicize their success against the American invasion.

Many of the best snipers were Chechen foreign mercenaries, making it even more difficult to locate a central command (it was the Chechnyans who joined forces against the Americans in Afghanistan, and Chechen brothers who were radicalized and bombed the Boston Marathon). Stephen's captain was on a rooftop, surrounded by several other marines and talking into his radio when the sniper shot him in the head from eight hundred meters away. Stephen was splashed by some of the blood and brain. As he mentioned this to me, he stared straight with a puzzled facial expression.

The troops often traveled as a convoy, and when they stopped, the soldiers hopped out and inspect the area for roadside bombs. The sides of the roads were strewn with trash. One Iraqi would set the bomb, another would set up the explosive device, and a third would go by and cover it with trash. And from a short distance, the area would be under video surveillance by those hoping to catch a kill. The IED batteries could last months, and it was difficult to get adequate intelligence. The US soldiers tortured suspected terrorists, but the information they gave about bomb caches was still frequently wrong. The toll of all this had been great on Stephen. He had once shot a suspected bomber who was standing fifteen feet away. "You just did that sort of thing," he explained.

Another time, his best friend, Jeff, hopped out of the Humvee and was hit in the back, and the bullet passed through the front, just below his chest, leaving a fatal gaping hole in his abdomen. "The next day his seat in the Humvee was empty—you notice these things." Stephen recalled, helplessly looking on, and asked me if I've heard if people can survive that sort of thing. I couldn't tell if he meant Jeff or himself.

Stephen remained concerned. "Sometimes we would talk about the violence like we talk about video games. But it's not the same. When it's real, there is a smell of blood and fear. They say it's getting better, but it will take ten years to get as good as it was before the invasion. There are some things we just can't fix." I knew he was right and hoped he was wrong, as I gave him an order for some tests and antacid medication.

Some of the wounds of the returning veterans are easy to see, while others lurk beneath the surface. The physician has the responsibility to treat the external as well as the internal wounds. This has become more difficult as we have trouble finding the time to dig out the stories, which contain the root of the problem. For the returning veterans, the care is limited, with a VA system unable to provide enough skilled therapists and programs to benefit these young returning soldiers and a health-care system geared to treat a very different kind of patient, not one bewildered and still fighting.

INTERNATIONAL

There has been increasing attention given to terrorism, so much so that it's difficult to gain a perspective that is not steeped in political agenda. Manipulated like rats in a Skinner box with the response patterned on Pavlov's research, we are expected to respond to the word *terrorism* with a fear response in order to generate either a vote or a contribution. We are extremely well informed about fear and ill informed about what to do in order to handle both fear and the terrorist threat. It reminds me of the line I once read that we're like eunuchs discussing the Kama Sutra. It was with that in mind that I decided to take my first trip to Israel in the fall of 2002. A group of American doctors had been organized in order to study the Israeli response to terrorism. It was easy to get a flight—not much competition to fly to Israel in those days.

When I arrived at customs in Tel Aviv, I was astonished that the agent knew that I was going to the conference in Jerusalem simply by checking my passport. I thought that was incredible security, and indeed, I felt very secure, but she informed me that it was simply the first conference in Israel in two years and everyone knew it. They were hoping it was a harbinger for more visits and, thus, more business. I immediately felt less secure.

We boarded a bus manned by an armed driver and an armed guard (not entirely reassuring). As we rode to Jerusalem, the driver pointed up a hill and announced, "That's where John the Baptist's father used to live." I asked the fellow seated next to me if I'd heard correctly, and we both smiled about that obscure bit of history and how unusual it was to make the connection between a two-thousand-year-old prominent Jewish family and modern Israel. It occurred to me that the next sight might be the hill where Moses's niece once had a party.

The driver then informed us that we would head directly to Hadassah Hospital for a visit. We were grubby, tired, and hungry and just wanted to get to the hotel, shower, and nap. But in response to our grumbling, the driver explained to us that there had been a suicide bombing earlier that day, and we were to visit the survivors. No one refused to go. The bomber, having already taken his "martyr photo" (used as a "marketing" poster in the occupied territories) had walked from Bethlehem, waited at the last bus stop to assure a capacity crowd, and boarded before blowing himself up, killing eleven children and adults and wounding others. Survivors were scooped up by fast-acting emergency personnel and rushed to the hospital for treatment.

As we rode to the hospital, I thought about the phrase "wounding others," which resonates differently from the way it does in a newscast when you are on the way to see those wounded others. The bomber had been wearing explosives encased in sharp metal objects coated with rat poison (the blood thinner warfarin, which prevents wounds from clotting) to provide shrapnel with a special toxic effect. The most sought-after suicide bombers are those with hepatitis to disseminate the virus along with the other forms of destruction. Medical personnel are worried about HIV-positive blood being sprayed as well.

We were ushered into the hospital and immediately shown the X-ray of a fifteen-year-old girl who had survived but was in critical condition. Her body was filled with shrapnel, and the bomber's watch had embedded in her neck, transecting the carotid, the major artery to her brain. She had been pierced in hundreds of locations, all oozing due to the shrapnel laced with blood thinner. She'd been transfused dozens of blood units by the time we saw her, and the fluid load had almost doubled her body weight. This young girl, who was the same age as my daughter at that time, was comatose, on a ventilator, and in the intensive care unit next to other survivors including an Arab worker and a family of four, all of whom had been injured in the blast.

That same day, the father of the bomber was interviewed on television. He praised his son as a martyr. Shortly thereafter, the Israeli army razed his home, which was the response in those days (Saddam Hussein would give the family of suicide bombers twenty-five thousand dollars in compensation—the price of a life). That evening, the father, distraught about his home, developed an abnormal heart rhythm and went to Hadassah Hospital where some of the same doctors caring for the bomb survivors also treated him. When asked by some of our crowd how they could take care of "these people," the hospital director responded in his thick Israeli accent, "If not, we lose our integrity and our humanity."

Whatever one thinks of Middle East politics, the message should be deeply embedded, like shrapnel, in every health worker: our job is to care for patients without regard to any other philosophical concern. There is time later, over coffee, over drinks, over gravesites, to ponder all those other impossible issues.

TO DO GOOD

In March 2012, I took a week off from my practice in Boston and went to a remote village in Nicaragua in order to provide medical care to a community sorely lacking modern health care. A group of seven doctors, along with an acupuncturist, twelve nurses and nursing students, three medical students, four premed students, two public health students, a public health psychiatrist, a psychologist, a pharmacist, a management consultant, a health-care insurance executive, a journalist, an accountant, and an investment banker, arrived in Managua then boarded a bus for the three-hour ride to Matagalpa, which was a shadow of its former self since an earthquake years before. Matagalpa served as our base.

Early each morning, we traveled on a rickety school bus for two hours up a seemingly impassable pockmarked road into the mountains until we arrived at the nearly impenetrable village of El Castillo—a smattering of homes with dirt floors, wood-burning cooking ovens, and hammocks for sleep. There was a church and a small K–6 school, neither of which had electricity nor running water. The loo was a hole in concrete (bring your own toilet paper and hand rinse).

On the first day, the bus didn't make it. The differential fell out two miles from town, so we walked in under the welcoming banner that the town had prepared for our arrival. The bus was repaired in three days. In the meantime, alternate transportation was arranged in a clanging, bone-shattering truck like those carrying migrant workers, which in fact we were. On the last hot and dusty day, the repaired bus did not have enough fuel, because when the bus, angled up the mountain, tried to accelerate, it lacked enough gas to get into the engine. Eventually, large plastic containers, reeking of diesel fumes, were taken up and funneled into the tank as a crowd gathered to watch, laughing and smoking, while I envisioned a fireball erupting, bringing a magnificent light to the native population.

The church was to serve as the clinic, but first it was required that we remove the pews, build exam tables out of plywood and two-by-fours, and separate the "rooms" with shower curtains hanging from ropes strung across ceiling beams. The open windows provided our only light. Whenever a refreshing breeze blew through the church/clinic from the open windows and doorway, the shower curtains flew around like crazy and papers scattered. If we didn't grab them in time, they shot off into space. Potential patients stood outside, cordoned off from the church and waiting to be let in by a nurse who acted like a bouncer at a popular New York club. In the meantime, chickens ran all over the place, ignoring our bouncer.

Due to an intransient health ministry, under the auspices of a Sandinista government suspicious of American intervention, we were only permitted to take a very limited amount of supplies with us. Aside from testing blood sugar with a glucometer (it wasn't unusual to find patients with sugars running several hundred points over normal) and urine with test strips, we had no lab. Prior to the trip, it was my great fear that I would be unable to diagnose the exotic tropical diseases I expected to find in Central America. In particular, how would I ever diagnose worms without the benefit of a lab detecting ova and parasites in the stool?

Thus, I was alarmed when I encountered the first patient with gastrointestinal complaints. I went through the usual litany of questions about abdominal pain, location, duration, reduced appetite, change in bowel habits, fever, blood in the stool, and weight loss. Then I asked if she had noticed worms in her feces. "Yes," she answered, and she described the eight-to-ten-inch grayish white worms I thought I would never be able to diagnose. Aha! So that's how you diagnose worms in a third-world country—you ask the patient. We had albendazole in our makeshift pharmacy, and I provided the treatment, but I ultimately learned that every three months, a local health official walked miles through the distant villages and treated those with known worms. She informed us that she added metronidazole (for parasite infection) to those with complaints of diarrhea. This seemed quite practical in this remote area of limited resources and diagnostic tools. Glad I could be of help.

Over the week I would see multitudes of patients who would walk miles from surrounding villages. One old guy limped into the clinic with back pain. He had severe kyphoscoliosis and was blind in his right eye, which was a grayish white orb. When he was young, he suffered headaches and would wrap a rag around his head soaked with either gasoline or kerosene. Apparently, it once oozed into his right eye, blinding him. I gave him Tylenol for his pain.

Another fellow came in with a ruptured left thigh muscle, now balled up but painless, without any deleterious effect on his leg function. I noticed his right hand was a claw and asked him what happened. Forty years ago, he had been robbed, and the robber slashed his wrist with a machete. Medical treatment was a rag around the wrist, and since it didn't necrose and develop gangrene, he was left with an intact hand, albeit nonfunctional.

A woman brought in her mentally challenged, nonverbal yet fully developed twenty-two-year-old daughter who was reportedly vomiting. She stayed home with her thirteen-year-old brother while her mother worked every day. Her belly was unusually distended, and she had reported worms. I asked if she was pregnant, and the mother replied that she couldn't be because she was retarded. I chose not to treat worms and arranged for a pregnancy test at a distant clinic, not realizing that many obstacles would have to be overcome in order to get the test and treat the girl. It will never be done.

One boy with seizures came in. Most seizures in that region were due to neurocysticercosis (brain worms) and were treated with antiseizure medication. One would treat the worms if scans or study of spinal fluid proved positive, but no such tests were available.

Not all cases were so easy. One woman needed gallbladder surgery but couldn't afford the cost of the bus ride (if you ask me, they should pay you to ride those things), nor could she afford the cost of any housing near the hospital as she recuperated.

Another had clear angina. In the Boston suburbs, if someone comes in with the complaint of substernal chest pain with effort, radiating to their left arm and jaw, associated with diaphoresis, nausea, and lightheadedness, relieved by rest, you know they read the Internet, because no one presents with such a textbook constellation of symptoms. Not so in El Castille. When a fifty-year-old man told me those symptoms evolving over the past few weeks, occurring as he would machete coffee fields, I knew this was the real deal. However, we were in the middle of nowhere, and if he were to undergo cardiac catheterization and receive a coronary artery stent, then placed on Plavix and aspirin, how would he be monitored? His pulse sped up to eighty-six as I walked with him (although mine sped up to 190 in the dust and altitude), so I figured a beta-adrenergic blocker plus aspirin might be a good first step to protect his heart. It wasn't clear how well this would turn out.

I arranged follow-up in the nearest town, but we were gone in a week without access to treatment results. I encountered a man in his forties complaining of left arm weakness. His gait was shuffling and awkward, and his exam revealed typical findings of Parkinson's disease, which is rare in someone so young. The treatment is limited to medications or experimental intervention. The medications were difficult to obtain and required monitoring. Since I couldn't arrange that in one day, I asked him to return the following day, but he didn't.

I felt I had falsely raised both my hopes and those of the villagers. After our return, e-mails and Facebook comments were exchanged among the group about how fulfilling the trip was. Maybe something we did was beneficial, maybe not. Some of us felt very good.

It was a reminder to me that there is a distinct difference between feeling good as the doctor and doing good for the patient.

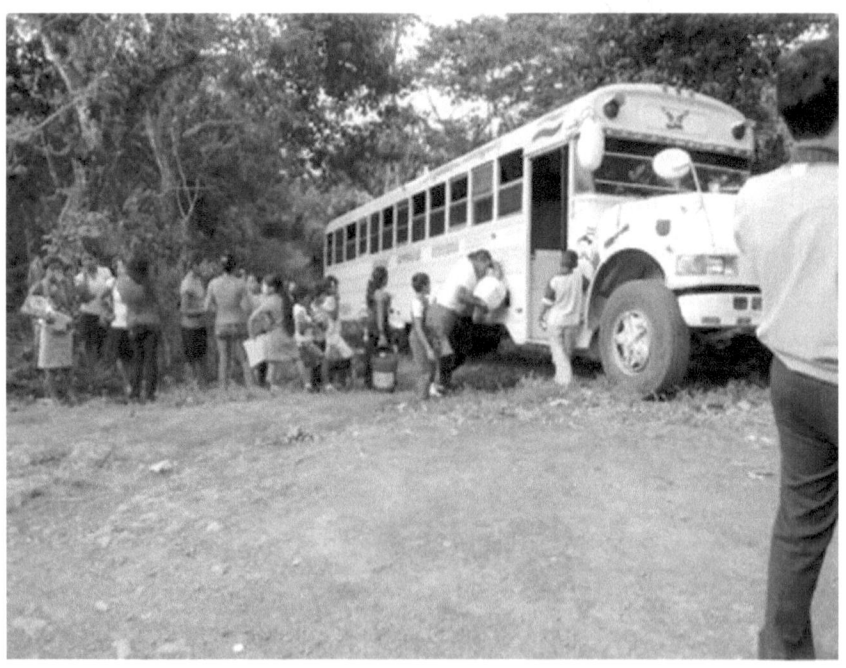

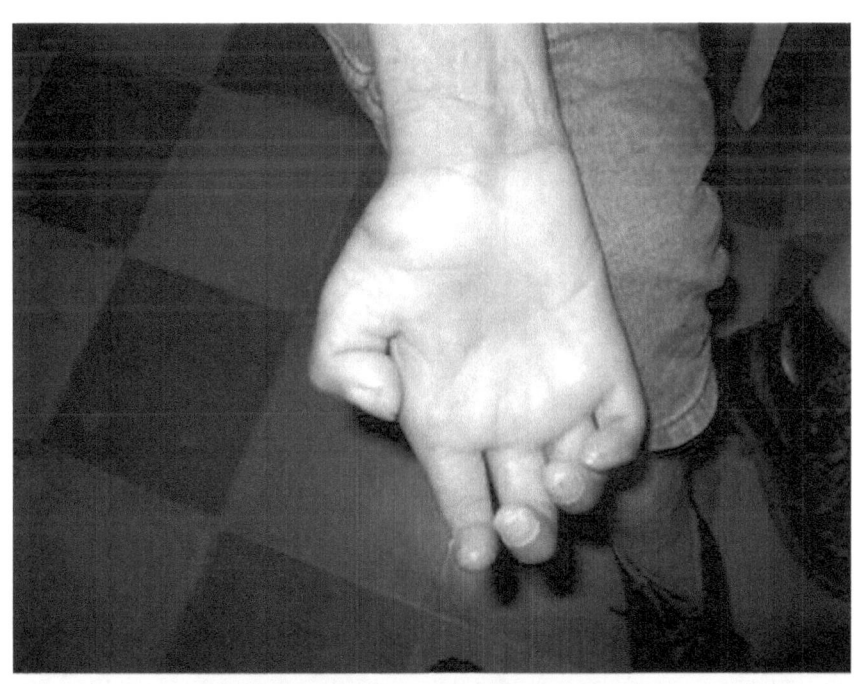
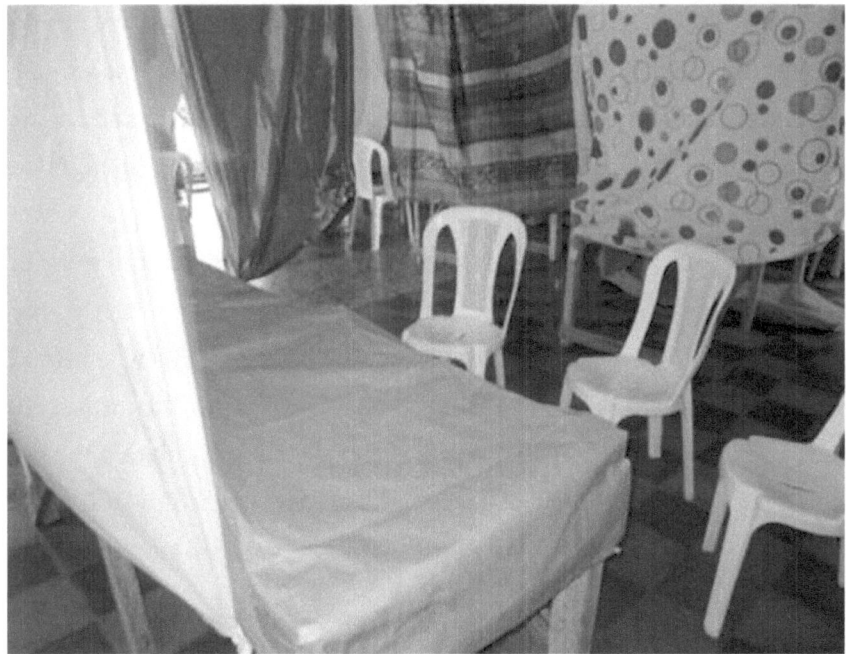

TRIP TO MEXICO

Haskel B. is not the sort of person you'd invite over for dinner. At eighty-nine, he is still a large man, heavyset, wobbly; he ambles like a bear. His hair is thin and gray, and most of his scalp is visible under those unkempt strands. Like Haskel, each hair had its own idea of where to go. He wears glasses, but they're greasy with one lens so cloudy that the eye on that side can't look out and, looking at him, one cannot see in. That doesn't seem to bother him much, because his eyes are not conjugate and view things differently even with clean lenses. His shirts are too small, often missing a button or popped open around his belly. His slacks are invariably stained and frayed. His hygiene leaves a lot to be desired. A lot.

As you can imagine, his behavior is odd. Doctors have placed him on a variety of medications in order to treat those oddities and get him out of their practice. I started seeing him twenty years ago shortly after he had visited Mexico. He was divorced and childless. His wife moved to Mexico just after she divorced him and made a new life for herself. Seventeen years after the divorce, Haskel boarded an airplane and flew down to Mexico and showed up at her door. She refused to let him in, so he returned home to Boston on the first available flight. That's the kind of guy he is.

Haskel isn't great about keeping medical appointments, and "continuity of care" isn't his thing. I wasn't remotely surprised when I heard he had fallen in his tiny, cluttered apartment and needed EMTs to pick him up, put him in an ambulance, and drive him to the emergency room. He was admitted to the hospital. That's when the trouble started. Once in the hospital, it was determined that muscles in his legs were so weak that he couldn't stand. It was also noted that the bones in his skull (examined because of the routine evaluation after a fall) revealed lytic lesions. We determined the problem to be multiple myeloma—a distinctly hideous cancer, which would probably kill him.

Since the workup and diagnosis progressed so quickly, and since it was determined that we had little to offer in the hospital, insurance payments were cut off. He still couldn't stand. I asked if he could go to rehab, but he had not satisfied the three-day requirement. "How about keeping him three days?" I asked the case manager. As usual, the response was, "No way—that costs the hospital money!" I fought the battle that I felt must be fought and was harassed by the case managers, the insurers, and the hospital administration (since they, too, had skin in the game).

It's hard to describe how awful this is for a doctor. Our mission, our job, our oath is to care for those in need of our services. We didn't sign on to care for the insurers, the computers, or the bottom line. However, that's what we're called upon to do by people who have no interest in those services and that oath—the Hippocratic Oath. I was informed by people with no connection to him (other than a fiscal interest) that Haskel had to leave. Haskel was probably informed as well, but Haskel was odd and might not have understood. Many, even those not so odd, wouldn't have understood. How does one understand a system that is supposed to provide for your welfare but refuses to? I was told that he must go home or go to rehab, but since he hadn't met the insurance requirements of three inpatient hospital days, he would have to pay "out of pocket" for rehab. And since he didn't have the money, he would have to go home. The problem was that Haskel couldn't walk. That was not the problem for the insurer, and it didn't seem to be the problem for the hospital. It was the problem for Haskel, and the problem for me. I argued (nothing new). The case managers worked behind my back and arranged for Haskel to go to rehab in spite of a less than three-day stay. I was amazed and complimented the case manager on the remarkable job she had done. Maybe I was too effusive, because she blushed. It wasn't until a day later that I learned Haskel had a great-nephew who was contacted by the case manager. He was told to cough up $5,000 for rehab or else Haskel would be sent home to die. He paid the money—the extorted money. That lasted a week before Haskel was sent home from rehab.

Haskel is confused about his situation. The insurer is happy, the hospital is happy, I am not happy.

OCTOPUS TRAP

It's a romantic notion "when two hearts beat as one," two people who have been together for so long that their hearts, like their lives, are entwined. Charlotte and Harold entered my office with matching walkers, each supporting the other, but neither able to make it alone. They communicated with chuckles, moans, and sighs, expressing to each other what no one listening nearby could possibly interpret. The electrons in the air seemed to allow for exchanges of messages between them. I'm not sure what else accounted for their communication. It was there even in silence.

Although over seventy, Harold maintained the cheerful nature of a man who can sell you a cheap suit and make you feel like Rockefeller. For many years after retiring from his job in clothing sales, Harold had suffered from an abnormal heart rhythm, and sometimes the electricity coursing through the heart would miss its connection and a heartbeat would be dropped. One evening, in 1993, his heart dropped several beats, and he fainted, prompting his wife to call 911. He was rushed to the hospital. While still at home, Charlotte (a woman who would compliment your shirt while ignoring the frayed collar so you'd feel good about yourself) felt "a sense of doom" and phoned me. As we spoke, I noticed she had difficulty completing sentences without pausing to catch her breath. She was not one to complain about her medical problems, but she felt something was very wrong. I arranged to meet her at the emergency room (where her husband had just arrived).

By the time I saw her, I noted a blue tinge to her lips and nail beds as she struggled to catch air. Her lungs had filled with fluid, and her blood pressure had dropped so low that she was in cardiogenic shock secondary to failure of the heart to pump enough blood to the rest of her tissues. Without immediate intervention, Charlotte would die. I stood by as the cardiologist performed an emergency cardiac catheterization to look carefully at her heart and repair any damage. Remarkably, the coronary arteries, which feed the heart, were normal, but Charlotte's heart had a funny shape with a ballooning at the bottom and a narrowing at the top. Using medication and special cardioprotective techniques, we were able to keep her alive. Within a few days, Charlotte was back to normal. A repeat test of her heart revealed that it was fine. Harold received a pacemaker to correct his abnormal heart rhythm, and soon the couple reunited.

A year later, however, Harold's pacemaker malfunctioned, and he fainted again. This time, Charlotte accompanied her husband to the hospital. By the time they arrived, she had a recurrence of the same cardiac event as the previous year. Again, she was almost dead, and again, we discovered the abnormally shaped heart. She recovered completely within days. The couple, again reunited and content (albeit a bit more cautious), returned home, eventually becoming older, frailer, and frequent visitors to my office.

Since that time, I have run across numerous medical journal reports of "stressful situations" resulting in cardiogenic shock in people with otherwise "normal" hearts. These stressors include earthquakes, court appearances, surprise parties, car accidents, and tragic news. The hearts of these people look alike, and in Japan, they describe this as "takotsubo cardiomyopathy," named for the fishing pot with a narrow neck and wide base that is used to trap octopus. Once in the trap, the octopus relaxes and is unable to return to its thinner form, making escape impossible. That's the risk when "two hearts beat as one."

THE LAST TIME

In early February 2007 Matilda C., sweet and suffering from dementia, wearing only a flimsy nightgown, walked onto her front porch. It was 2:00 AM, and her husband, Lou, was still asleep. She was discovered outside when the police arrived in response to the missing-person call from Lou at seven in the morning. The police knew the address well; this was not the first time that Lou had called them, but it was the last time. Matilda was found laid out on the porch, in a hypothermic coma. She was rushed to the hospital, and her core body temperature was down about sixteen degrees, from a normal of 98.6 to 82 degrees Fahrenheit (not a bad temperature for summer, but potentially deadly for a core temperature).

By the time she was evaluated in the hospital, Matilda's muscle enzymes and potassium levels were elevated, and she had abnormal clotting due to toxic effects of the cold. Her electrocardiogram revealed ominous rhythms and Osborn waves, indicating severe hypothermia. The emergency team administered heated nebulizers, which warmed the largest surface area—the lung alveoli (the thousands of small air sacs in the lung account for an enormous area, which is readily accessed by inhaling heated air). Additionally, the staff administered heated intravenous fluids and warming blankets. Careful attention was paid to cardiac and kidney function. She survived.

Due to her dementia, she was placed in a nursing home. Although Lou understood the need for this move, he wanted to be admitted to the same facility with her. He felt lost without her as she was lost without him; in sixty-two years of marriage, they were rarely apart. He was upset when informed there were no available male beds at that time, and Lou was denied admission to that particular nursing home. In sorrow or in stress over the ensuing months, he had a heart attack. It wasn't his first. Over the years, his heart muscle had been damaged so many times that it was scarred down and was only pumping at one-quarter capacity. This particular time, Lou's recovery was taking longer than usual. He was still in the hospital on a lovely spring day when Matilda was taken for a walk on the grounds around the nursing home, which had become her permanent residence. Following her walk, she sat down in a large stuffed chair in the nursing home lobby. It was there that she suffered a cardiac arrest. Emergency personnel resuscitated her and took her to a nearby hospital (about five miles away from where Lou was hospitalized) where she died.

Meanwhile, Lou was in rapidly failing health. That same day, he slipped into a coma. With input from Lou and Matilda's children, I decided to withhold aggressive treatment. We would allow him to pass away without further therapy and, since the end was near, decided to keep him in his bed in the hospital to avoid the indignity of a chaotic transfer to a nursing home where he would either die in transit or upon arrival.

This commonsense approach used to be the standard in medical care. In our present health-care system, this sort of decision sets off a bureaucratic shuffle in which the case managers (hospital employees driven by insurance rules to minimize losses to the insurer) try to hustle the patient out to a nursing home in an attempt to save money for the hospital (which has been forced to play by these draconian rules in order to make a profit). This standoff created a heated exchange between the case managers and me. The already-grieving family was overwhelmed. The hospital chaplain was called in by one of the nurses caring for Lou to lend a degree of moral imperative.

Not surprisingly, prior to any final resolution of the quarrel, Lou died, almost exactly twenty-four hours after his wife died. His children said that she called him from the grave, and they were relieved. The case manager skulked away to assign value to another life, and the distraught chaplain approached me to ask, "Why couldn't we avoid a confrontation over the health-care dollar as a family is grieving and a patient is dying? What have we become?"

THE TRAP?

Whom should we treat, and whom should we neglect? It seems an extraordinarily inappropriate question. Yet doctors are faced with just that dilemma. There seems to be plenty of room for more humanity, and we stand to learn much of it from our patients. The problem is that barriers erected by insurers as well as certain technologies inhibit the doctor-patient interaction. Everyone would like to be listened to without the risk of an administrator or a computer interpreting the narrative.

There is a challenge for the doctor when a bond with the patient gets too tight. The relationship with the patient gives us satisfaction, but it takes a little bit from us as well. Some doctors are fearful that clinical distance from the patient may be breached by collecting an excess of personal and historical information by listening too much too intently. The present greed-soaked insurance-centered system offers a solution: bureaucrats determine care and require that the interaction gets immediately put into a computer; the interface is with a computer screen as the doctor clicks information on the screen, which prevents the doctor from looking at the patient. Naturally, a system whereby medical information is sent via computer is a wonderful concept. Unfortunately, the fact that there is little privacy with these systems has been ignored or brushed aside as if personal medical information is the same as information found on Facebook. Currently most labs and technological studies (such as X-rays) are available to physicians on computer systems, which is great. Medication use and drug interactions are also important ways for computers to aid physicians. But the present computerized system is not universal, thus preventing information sharing between different insurance networks, yet it permits an insurer to screen records, to limit procedures and prescriptions, and eventually to adjust premiums and coverage, as well as potentially collecting information about costly individual patient-lifestyle decisions, which is the incentive for insurance funding of the "electronic medical record." It results in distancing the physician from the patient while it tightens the bond between the patient and the insurer. As Justice Harlan Stone once said about law, and what I now feel is true of medicine, corporate power "has made the learned profession of an earlier day the obsequious servant of business, and tainted it with the morals and manners of the marketplace in its most anti-social manifestations."

When I try to use electronic records, I notice an immediate mind shift. Over the thirty years I've been in practice, I've developed a method of focusing on the patient. The moment I see them, I recall the basics of their medical problems (that case of babesiosis ten years ago, the heart attack three years ago) and bits of life information (the granddaughter with leukemia, the son with drug abuse)—I know who they are. It's a habit that evolved to the point that it is a "hardwired" circuit in my brain. It is supplemented by facts in the record. However, the moment that I try to put information into an electronic medical record, my focus changes. After all, the computer is interesting, and it leads me into different "wormholes" similar to a video game. When I look at the computer, I feel my brain click from the focus on the patient to focus upon the computer, and I can't seem to stop it.

So, for now, I have returned to a written chart with the computer as a supplement, not a replacement. I have spoken with many physicians about this, and they share my concern. It's such a common complaint that it prompted a letter from a doctor/administrator who stated that in order to make the doctor interaction feel more personal, consider adding a computer popup such as, "How is that new puppy?" or "How was the vacation?" This can be accomplished by staring at the screen with an occasional glance in the direction of the patient. The gulf between the doctor and patient is further widened by discouraging doctors from caring for their patients in the hospital. Instead a sick patient is assigned a hospital doctor called a hospitalist. The hospitalist service changes almost as often as the medical team of interns and residents changes. The June 2007 *New England Journal of Medicine* had an article noting that for a five-day hospital stay, there is an average of fifteen handoffs between different doctors, thus assuring no continuity as no one really knows the patient well. What's expedient may not be worth the human sacrifice (recall the lesson of Agamemnon, who traded his daughter's life for a good breeze).

When I drop my shirts off at the dry cleaners, they say, "Hello, Mr. Terry." (My wife's first name is Terry.) The dry cleaner knows me, but if I were sick and wound up on the hospitalist service, the doctor caring for me would know me less well than my dry cleaner. Sure, it's easier not to worry about the tightening of a bond, as in the "Octopus Trap," but it does not serve either the patient or the doctor well. What are we losing? What have we lost? I don't really care if my dry cleaning is that personal, but I definitely want my health care to be most personal. I feel it's necessary to offer my patients personalized care. I am always surprised, though I shouldn't be, when they brighten the moment I enter their hospital room. After all, I've learned that getting to know the person, and not just the patient, contributes to the healing process. The patient wants the bond. It presumes more personal and better care, and the doctor, at the heart of his training, must encourage it and be willing to enter the trap, allowing him to expand and to relax, because it's not just a trap; it's empathy, and it should be our job.

THE LAST WORD

The wait for first words can seem interminable, but last words come too soon. Sometimes, using information from those last words, the account moves backward. The movie *Citizen Kane* was based on investigating the protagonist's last word: *rosebud*. That story recounted a life based upon a search for the meaning of that word. Words are welcome during the final days of life; they are especially poignant. Not everyone can sum things up with humor and panache as Oscar Wilde did with his last words: "Either that wallpaper goes, or I do!" But often, the last words make a point and, perhaps, complete a life story. We use the stories of others to think about our own lives—many parts are skipped, and many more are forgotten. It is the fortunate few who are given a chance to review those memories and to share them with others in a final attempt to reach that moment when things are clarified, to recall it before it is entirely forgotten, passed into the vapor that was once our spot. Maybe those last words will help get things right in the end.

An eighty-three-year-old Jewish man tripped and fell in his Chicago apartment, contusing his spinal cord. This resulted in quadriplegia, leaving him unable to move his arms or legs and relegating him to a bed and a special motorized wheelchair. He was intelligent, articulate, and feisty, but the injury left him tragically impaired, leaving only a wisp of his essence. His left hand was permanently flexed into a palsied grasp, occasionally twitching while he would listen to conversations. That grasping hand seemed to attempt to hold sound or memories before they passed. He spoke less and less, and when he did, it was in whispers due to his generalized weakness. He had been moved from his apartment to a long-term-care nursing facility. Whenever I visited, he would brighten, and whenever I departed, he would whisper, "Do you have to go? Don't. Please. Oh, that's okay. Good-bye." The last time I left, however, when I said "I have to go," he remained mute. I asked, "Aren't you going to say good-bye?" Looking directly at me with sky-blue eyes under heavy lids, he still didn't speak. I asked again. This time he whispered something inaudible. I put my ear to his lips and asked him to repeat it. It was soft and muffled, sounding like "Gefffssish." I urged him to repeat it yet again. It sounded the same, "Geffefffissh." I said, "Are you saying gefilte fish?" He grinned and nodded yes.

Gefilte fish is an odd sort of fish and matzo meal mixture primarily eaten on Passover, which is the joyful and instructive ceremony recalling the Jewish liberation from slavery and eventual exodus from Egypt. That exodus had occurred more than three thousand years ago and remains a focal point in Jewish tradition. A typical Passover meal starts with gefilte fish. A couple of generations ago, it was common to make this dish in your home, but after a few stories of women coming down with fish tapeworm (*Diphyllobothrium latum*), stores began selling more and more gefilte fish in jars and cans, and home preparation declined. But consumption of gefilte fish remained high.

Every year at Passover, Jewish families gather to read about the history of the exodus from Egypt. Information is passed from the old to the young. As part of the celebration, food is consumed, wine is drunk, and songs are sung. Strangers are invited as guests to share the meal. The Passover meal remains meaningful as a source of history and ethics, decrying slavery and praising personal integrity—a reminder that the weak and infirm need an advocate, a protector with a special skill... to part the waters. Passover has occurred annually for a couple of millennia. Its importance remains in community celebration, speaking truth to power and teaching right from wrong.

Some people love gefilte fish, some hate it, and all have an opinion about it. "Gefilte fish!" I responded. "You said gefilte fish. I too prefer it to good-bye. If I never see you again, and those are the last words you ever say to me, I'm fine with that. In fact, I'm really quite comfortable with that." At that moment, my father grinned again, and I walked away to catch my plane back to Boston.

www.ingramcontent.com/pod-product-compliance
Lightning Source LLC
Chambersburg PA
CBHW030944180526
45163CB00002B/694